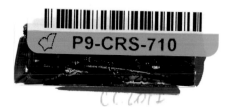

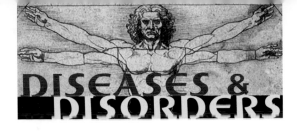

MRSA

Titles in the Diseases and Disorders series include:

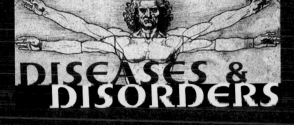

DISEASES & DISORDERS

MRSA

Barbara Sheen

LUCENT BOOKS
A part of Gale, Cengage Learning

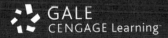
GALE
CENGAGE Learning

Detroit • New York • San Francisco • New Haven, Conn • Waterville, Maine • London

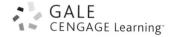
GALE
CENGAGE Learning·

LIBRARY OF CONGRESS CATALOGING-IN-PUBLICATION DATA

Sheen, Barbara.
 MRSA / by Barbara Sheen.
  p. cm. -- (Diseases and disorders)
 Includes bibliographical references and index.
 ISBN 978-1-4205-0144-5 (hardcover)
 1. Staphylococcus aureus infections. I. Title.
 RC116.S8S45 2010
 616.9'2--dc22

2009032644

Lucent Books
27500 Drake Rd.
Farmington Hills, MI 48331

ISBN-13: 978-1-4205-0144-5
ISBN-10: 1-4205-0144-5

Printed in the United States of America
1 2 3 4 5 6 7 13 12 11 10 09

Printed by Bang Printing, Brainerd, MN, 1st Ptg., 10/2009

Table of Contents

FOREWORD

"The Most Difficult Puzzles Ever Devised"

Charles Best, one of the pioneers in the search for a cure for diabetes, once explained what it is about medical research that intrigued him so. "It's not just the gratification of knowing one is helping people," he confided, "although that probably is a more heroic and selfless motivation. Those feelings may enter in, but truly, what I find best is the feeling of going toe to toe with nature, of trying to solve the most difficult puzzles ever devised. The answers are there somewhere, those keys that will solve the puzzle and make the patient well. But how will those keys be found?"

Since the dawn of civilization, nothing has so puzzled people—and often frightened them, as well—as the onset of illness in a body or mind that had seemed healthy before. A seizure, the inability of a heart to pump, the sudden deterioration of muscle tone in a small child—being unable to reverse such conditions or even to understand why they occur was unspeakably frustrating to healers. Even before there were names for such conditions, even before they were understood at all, each was a reminder of how complex the human body was, and how vulnerable.

6

While our grappling with understanding diseases has been frustrating at times, it has also provided some of humankind's most heroic accomplishments. Alexander Fleming's accidental discovery in 1928 of a mold that could be turned into penicillin has resulted in the saving of untold millions of lives. The isolation of the enzyme insulin has reversed what was once a death sentence for anyone with diabetes. There have been great strides in combating conditions for which there is not yet a cure, too. Medicines can help AIDS patients live longer, diagnostic tools such as mammography and ultrasounds can help doctors find tumors while they are treatable, and laser surgery techniques have made the most intricate, minute operations routine.

This "toe-to-toe" competition with diseases and disorders is even more remarkable when seen in a historical continuum. An astonishing amount of progress has been made in a very short time. Just two hundred years ago, the existence of germs as a cause of some diseases was unknown. In fact, it was less than 150 years ago that a British surgeon named Joseph Lister had difficulty persuading his fellow doctors that washing their hands before delivering a baby might increase the chances of a healthy delivery (especially if they had just attended to a diseased patient)!

Each book in Lucent's Diseases and Disorders series explores a disease or disorder and the knowledge that has been accumulated (or discarded) by doctors through the years. Each book also examines the tools used for pinpointing a diagnosis, as well as the various means that are used to treat or cure a disease. Finally, new ideas are presented—techniques or medicines that may be on the horizon.

Frustration and disappointment are still part of medicine, for not every disease or condition can be cured or prevented. But the limitations of knowledge are being pushed outward constantly; the "most difficult puzzles ever devised" are finding challengers every day.

A Growing Problem

In January 2005 Peg McQueary nicked her ankle while shaving. It was a tiny cut, but that little opening in her skin provided a perfect entry point for dangerous bacteria. Two weeks later McQueary developed a pus-filled boil on her ankle. Shortly thereafter, her leg swelled to three times its normal size. It was hot, tender, and painful.

McQueary went to see her doctor. He rushed her to the hospital, where she was intravenously administered vancomycin, a powerful antibiotic. It took more than a month for McQueary's leg to heal.

Three years later, McQueary still has problems. She is plagued with recurring infections and continuous pain in her leg. "My case," she says, "is not much different than thousands of others."[1]

McQueary had an invasive methicillin-resistant *Staphylococcus aureus* (MRSA) infection. It is a bacterial infection that can cause a wide array of problems, ranging from minor skin irritations to life-threatening conditions. MRSA differs from most other bacterial infections because it is resistant to many antibiotics. This makes it difficult to treat and, therefore, more dangerous than other bacterial infections. It is also very contagious.

MRSA is the cause of millions of infections annually. According to the Centers for Disease Control and Prevention (CDC), approximately 12 million people visit health care facilities in the United States for suspected MRSA infections each year. In 2005 alone, MRSA infections were the leading cause of soft-tissue infections in hospital emergency rooms.

Although most MRSA infections are noninvasive and thus not serious, invasive MRSA infections, like McQueary's, can be deadly. They strike about 94,000 Americans annually and cause about 19,000 deaths. That is more than HIV/AIDS, which causes about 12,500 deaths each year.

A New Condition

MRSA infections are relatively new. They were first identified in patients of hospitals and nursing homes during the 1960s. MRSA infections started to be found among otherwise healthy individuals outside of a health care setting during the late 1990s.

A MRSA infection can start out as a minor skin irritation, like a cut from a razor, and turn into a serious illness.

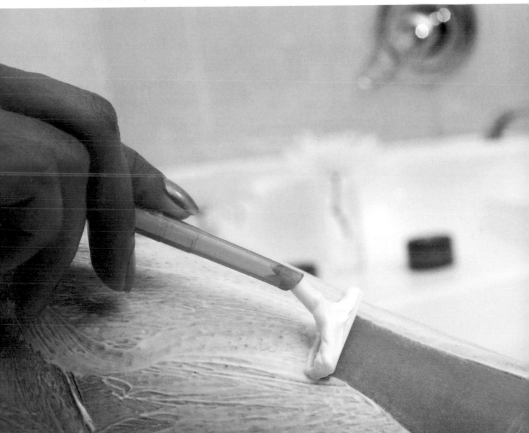

In a short period of time, MRSA infections have skyrocketed. The CDC has been tracking MRSA cases in nine states for more than thirty years. Their records show that MRSA infections accounted for only 2 percent of all *Staphylococcus aureus* (staph or *S. aureus*) infections in 1974. That number rose to 22 percent by 1995. It shot up to almost 65 percent by 2008 and is still rising. A 2007 American Medical Association study found that 46 out of every 1,000 hospitalized patients in the United States have a MRSA infection. Of these, approximately 32 patients per 100,000 have the invasive variety.

Because the number of MRSA cases is increasing so rapidly, the infections are so hard to treat, and the death toll is mounting. Scott Fridkin, a medical epidemiologist at the CDC, warns that MRSA "is a significant public health problem."[2]

MRSA cases are also growing worldwide. Five years ago Canada, Germany, Greece, and Spain reported almost no MRSA infections. They are now seeing more and more cases. In Greece, 48.6 percent of all staph infections are now due to MRSA, as are 27.2 percent in Germany and 23.5 percent in Spain. In England, the incidence of invasive MRSA infections tripled between 1997 and 2004, going from 2,422 cases to 7,684. Elizabeth Bancroft, a medical epidemiologist at the Los Angeles County Department of Health Services, describes the growing threat MRSA poses both nationally and internationally in this way: "This bug has gone from 0 to 60, not in five seconds but in almost five years. It spreads by contact, so if it gets into a community that is fairly close-knit, that's all it needs to be passed."[3]

The Costs to Individuals and Society

As MRSA infections become more common, the cost to individuals and society rises. Many MRSA patients face physical and emotional challenges, along with economic problems like lost wages and medical expenses.

MRSA also presents financial issues for society. The cost of treating hospitalized individuals with MRSA is about $4 billion a year. That is approximately triple the cost of treating patients with the same diagnosis who do not develop an infection. The

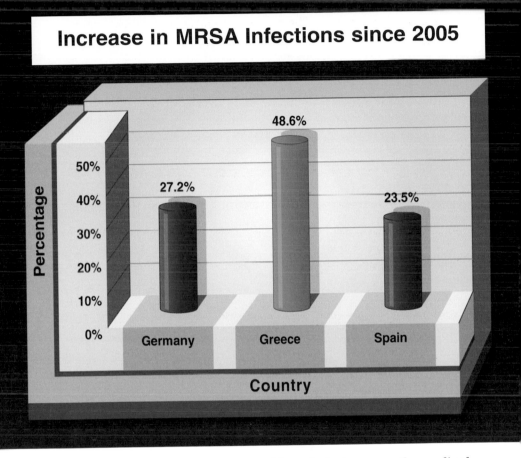

Increase in MRSA Infections since 2005

higher cost is due to prolonged hospital stays, costly medical procedures, and medications.

A 2008 study by the Pfizer Corporation found that patients with MRSA are hospitalized an average of ten days longer than patients with non-MRSA infections. The resulting cost ranges from $27,083 to $34,900 per case. Patients, insurance companies, the government, and taxpayers pay these costs. Hospitals are also economically burdened by these infections, which cut into their profits. An article on the Web site of the Committee to Reduce Infection Deaths explains:

Infections erode hospital profits, because rarely are hospitals paid fully for the added weeks or months of care when a patient gets an infection. For example, Allegheny General Hospital in Pittsburgh would have made a profit treating a 37-year-old video programmer and father of four who was admitted with acute pancreatitis, but the economics changed when the patient developed a MRSA bloodstream infection. He had to stay in the hospital 86 days, and the hospital lost $41,813, according to research by Richard Shannon, a former chairman of the Department of Medicine at Allegheny.[4]

The Need for Awareness

These figures are especially disturbing because there are simple steps, such as cleaning and covering wounds, not sharing personal items, and frequent hand washing, that can help prevent MRSA infections. Unfortunately, there is limited knowledge of the illness and its potential problems. As a result, many individuals do not seek treatment until the illness has caused significant damage to their bodies. Moreover, because MRSA infections are relatively new, many health care professionals do not test for the condition.

Learning more about the illness, its causes and symptoms, and how it is transmitted can help inhibit its spread. It can also help individuals to seek prompt and effective treatment, which can save their lives. MRSA education and prevention advocate Christina Jones explains:

> I am not in the medical profession, in fact, I am just a regular lay person, who has come to learn the hard way a great deal about something that I wish I never had to know about. My husband nearly died last year of a bacterial infection called MRSA. I want to be sure that our community is informed about MRSA because it is so prevalent across the United States, and so few people become aware of it before it directly affects their lives. . . . MRSA can be dealt with easily, without panic, by avoiding it in the first place, but we cannot fight that of which we are unaware. . . . What you don't know CAN hurt you. In fact, it can kill you.[5]

CHAPTER ONE

What Is MRSA?

Methicillin-resistant *Staphylococcus aureus* (MRSA) is the name given to a strain of the *Staphylococcus aureus* bacteria that is resistant to a number of antibiotics. MRSA bacteria are relatively harmless unless they gain entry into the body, where they can cause serious damage. MRSA infections are easily spread. Anyone can contract the condition. Some individuals, however, are at greater risk.

Invisible Microorganisms

Bacteria are single-celled microorganisms too small to be seen without a microscope. They are found everywhere, including in and on the human body. Some forms of bacteria are harmful, but other types are harmless. In fact, some types of harmless bacteria are used to make vaccines and medicines. Other types help the body to function by taking up space in the body that would otherwise serve as colonization sites for more dangerous bacteria. These bacteria outnumber human body cells ten to one.

Other forms of bacteria are not as useful. They produce harmful chemicals or toxins that attack the body. *Staphylococcus aureus* falls into this group.

A Superbug

About one in three individuals are colonized with or carry small quantities of *Staphylococcus aureus* on their skin, groin, armpits, and/or in their noses and throats. One in ten carries methicillin-resistant *Staphylococcus aureus*. In most cases, these bacterial colonies are harmless. Many of these colonies are too small to cause any damage. And, because *S. aureus* is not a good competitor, it is unable to displace helpful bacteria in order to gain a stronghold. Staph colonies become dangerous

Staphylococcus aureus secretes powerful toxins that destroy host cells in a variety of ways, thus deserving the name "superbug."

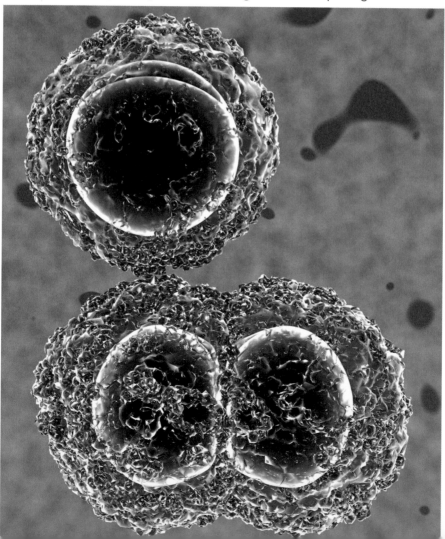

when an initiating event, such as a break in the skin, occurs; this then provides the bacteria a portal of entry into the body.

Once inside the body, *Staphylococcus aureus* secretes powerful toxins, which attack and destroy host cells, converting them into nutrients for bacterial growth. As the bacteria multiply, more and more toxins are released. Some of these toxins break down internal tissue, which allows the bacteria to enter the bloodstream. Once in the bloodstream, the toxins can destroy disease-fighting white blood cells, break apart red blood cells, cause the formation of blood clots, attack the top layer of skin, and, eventually, harm every organ in the body. Because of these factors, scientists and health care professionals often refer to *S. aureus* as a "superbug." According to Michael Otto of the National Institute of Allergy and Infectious Diseases, "Different bacteria have different strategies to attack the human immune system. S. aureus seems to have a lot of strategies, it's really good at that."[6]

The extent of the damage *S. aureus* causes depends on how far the infection spreads and the strength of the affected individual's immune system. Generally, the infection remains localized in the skin around the point of entry, causing boils and cellulitis, or swelling and tenderness of the skin and underlying tissue.

The longer the bacteria remain untreated, however, the more the infection grows and the more likely it is to spread throughout the body. Infectious disease expert Bertha S. Ayi explains that a *Staphylococcus aureus* colony

> can be likened to an armed enemy who moved uncomfortably close next door or came to live in your basement purely for the reason that he was homeless and needed a place to stay. All along you knew he owned weapons that could harm you, but he seemed pleasant most of the time and never expressed any intent to hurt you. These weapons could potentially be used to break down the walls of your house and allow entry into your personal space. The enemy in the sense is Staph aureus and the weapons are the toxins and chemicals that the bug could use to invade your skin, multiply, and cause disease.[7]

A Dangerous Mutation

S. aureus bacteria, like all forms of bacteria, are constantly mutating. In order to survive, bacteria evolve, producing newer, stronger strains. There are many different strains of *S. aureus*. Some strains produce more toxins, and some are more susceptible to antibiotics. Therefore, some strains are more dangerous than others. MRSA is one of the most dangerous forms of *S. aureus*.

Before the discovery of antibiotics, even a localized staph infection was often a death sentence. The widespread use of antibiotics changed that. Antibiotics work by killing off weak bacteria. Some bacteria, however, survive. These bacteria mutate, forming a stronger strain of bacteria that is better able to resist the antibiotics. So, although antibiotics are necessary to fight a bacterial infection, exposure to the drugs encourages the development of antibiotic-resistant bacteria. For instance, penicillin kills bacteria by binding to the bacteria's cell walls. Penicillin-resistant bacteria, like MRSA, contain a mutant gene that manufactures a protein that makes it impossible for penicillin to bind to the bacteria.

S. aureus is especially good at changing. Only four years after penicillin was mass-produced, a strain of *S. aureus* appeared that could resist the drug. This new strain of *S. aureus* was treated with other penicillin-like drugs. Over time, the bacteria developed the ability to resist a large class of antibiotics known as beta-lactams. These drugs include methicillin and other penicillin-like antibiotics as well as a group of antibiotics known as cephalosporins. This strain, which is known as methicillin-resistant *Staphylococcus aureus*, is what causes MRSA infections. It is resistant to fifteen to thirty different antibiotics. This means doctors have few medications available to effectively treat it.

Making matters worse, MRSA—like all forms of bacteria—is constantly changing. As a result, new strains of MRSA keep appearing that are resistant to even more antibiotics. One particular strain is resistant to vancomycin, which is one of the only antibiotics that is effective in treating severe MRSA infections.

According to Chip Chambers, chief of the Infectious Disease Division at San Francisco General Hospital:

> We may eventually lose what drugs we do have, and that is a real concern in treating MRSA. . . . This organism-type of bacteria is very adept at adapting to any antibiotic that we throw at it. . . . From the bacteria point of view, antibiotics are the biggest problem they've had to face in their evolution and they're doing a good job of adapting.[8]

MRSA Bacteria Spread Easily

Besides being resistant to multiple antibiotics, MRSA infections are extremely contagious. Individuals with an active infection and those who carry the bacteria can transmit the disease. Skin-to-skin contact with an infected wound or bacterial colony passes the bacteria from person to person. Infected and colonized individuals can also pass the bacteria to objects. Computer keyboards, desktops and countertops, telephones, gym equipment, doorknobs, medical equipment, locker room floors, blankets, towels, and clothes are just a few of the thousands of items that can harbor the bacteria, which can survive for about two months on hard and soft surfaces. Touching contaminated objects passes the germs along.

Most people are unaware that they have come in contact with the bacteria. When it is transmitted onto an individual's skin, it forms a harmless colony. These newly colonized people become carriers. They can inadvertently spread the bacteria to other individuals by direct and indirect contact. The cycle can continue indefinitely. Carriers will only develop an infection if the bacteria gain entry into their bodies.

The Washington State Department of Health warns:

> If you have an active MRSA infection on your skin, it is contagious. If someone touches your infections, or touches something that came in contact with your infection (like a towel), that person could get MRSA. If you are a MRSA carrier, you still have the bacteria on your skin and in your nose. If you don't wash your hands properly, things that you use or touch with your hands can give the

bacteria to other people. MRSA can also be found in the liquid that comes out of your nose or mouth when you cough or sneeze. Remember, if you have MRSA it is possible to spread it to family, friends, other people close to you, and even to pets.[9]

Hospital-Acquired MRSA Infections

There are two distinct types of MRSA. Each has a slightly different genetic makeup. To categorize the type of the bacteria and how the condition is spread, MRSA infections are classified as either hospital-acquired or community-acquired MRSA infections (HA-MRSA or CA-MRSA).

As the name implies, hospital-acquired MRSA infections are contracted in hospitals or other health care facilities, such as nursing homes. The infection may appear while the patient is hospitalized or after he or she has been released. HA-MRSA strains are usually resistant not only to beta-lactams but also to other types of antibiotics. Because many hospitalized patients are weak and their immune systems are compromised, HA-MRSA infections are often quite serious. Six out of ten blood infections in patients in intensive care units in the United States are HA-MRSA infections.

Ironically, HA-MRSA infections often present a greater risk to patients than the original condition for which they were hospitalized. In one HA-MRSA case, a woman was admitted to the hospital with a broken shoulder. While hospitalized, she contracted a fatal MRSA infection that compromised her ability to breathe and move. It eventually caused her vital organs to fail. The patient's daughter recalls that her mother "walked into the hospital as a healthy, beautiful woman. But she wound up as a quadriplegic [someone whose arms and legs are paralyzed] on a ventilator. . . . I never could have dreamt something like this would happen. It was so pitiful."[10]

HA-MRSA constitutes an estimated 85 percent of all MRSA cases. Hospital patients often have open wounds, which provide perfect entrance points for MRSA. Invasive medical devices such as catheters can spread the bacteria and act as a carrier directly into the body. And, because the bacteria can

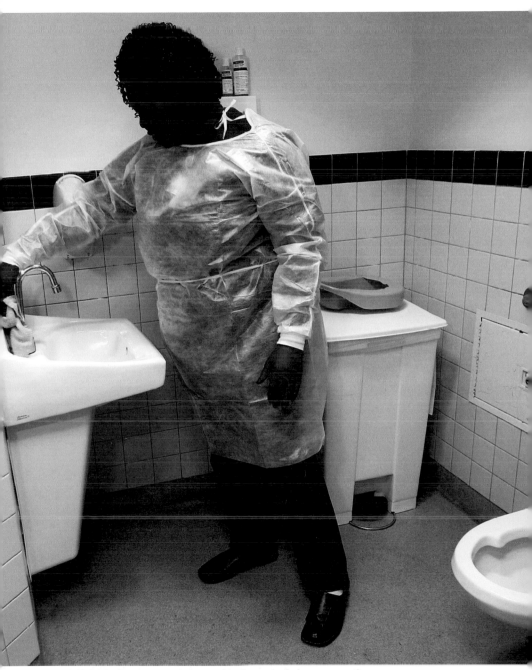

MRSA infections originated in hospitals because of cross-contamination. Now, staff are diligent to disinfect all surfaces, like this housekeeping worker at Miami VA Medical Center.

survive on so many surfaces for so long, one infected patient can contaminate hundreds of objects, including bedrails, wheelchairs, remote-control devices, stethoscopes, blood pressure cuffs, and other medical equipment. A 2003 study in a

Drug-Resistant Bacteria and the Improper Use of Antibiotics

There is no way to stop bacteria from becoming drug resistant. The improper use of antibiotics, however, accelerates the process.

Although viruses do not respond to antibiotics, they are often prescribed when patients insist on medication. Exposure to the drugs contributes to bacteria in the body mutating and developing drug resistance.

In the case of a bacterial infection, the failure to finish a full course of antibiotics causes trouble, too. Such action almost guarantees that bacteria, which have been exposed to the antibiotic, are left in the body to multiply and mutate. Christina Jones, a MRSA awareness advocate, explains what is happening:

> When you take antibiotics that you pressured your doctor to prescribe because you just felt horrible, even though you didn't have a bacterial infection, you have made the bacteria that were there stronger and more resistant to that antibiotic. When you have a bacterial infection and stop taking your prescribed antibiotics when you feel better, rather than completing the full course, you have made those bacteria that weren't killed off a little stronger and more resistant.

Christina Jones, "An Open Letter to My Community," MRSA Resources, September 20, 2005. www.mrsaresources.com/an-open-letter-to-my-community/.

hospital in Tours, France, found that 77 percent of the rolling blood pressure cuffs in the hospital and 63 percent of individual cuffs were infected with MRSA. Patients who come in contact with these objects can easily become infected.

Although hospital equipment and surfaces are routinely disinfected, many areas are missed. In 2007 researchers at Boston University examined forty-nine operating rooms in four area hospitals. They found that more than half of the surfaces in the operating rooms that could harbor MRSA were not disinfected.

In a follow-up study, the researchers examined patient rooms in twenty hospitals in the Northeast. Once again, more than half of the surfaces that should have been disinfected after patients were released were overlooked. A 2001 Japanese study looked at hospitals in Tokyo. The researchers found that when a nurse goes into the room of a patient with MRSA, even if the nurse has no physical contact with the patient but touches objects in the room, the nurse's gloves become contaminated 42 percent of the time.

A woman who contracted HA-MRSA after a hospital stay describes her experience:

> I had a lump removed from my side on Jan. 3, 2008. I had just returned to work when I came down with a fever at work and my incision site started to swell and [cause me] tremendous pain. . . . I was diagnosed with MRSA. Where I got it is anyone's guess (the operating room?). Did someone not wash their hands or was equipment infected? I may never know but now my husband packs my incision everyday and the pain is horrible. There is no telling when it will heal.[11]

Community-Acquired MRSA

Community-acquired MRSA is a recent development that first appeared in the late 1990s. According to infectious disease expert Hernan R. Chang, it strikes healthy individuals who

> have not had hospitalization or surgery, dialysis, residence in a long-term care facility, skilled nursing facility or hospice, during the past year; they have no permanent

indwelling catheters, . . . they have no medical history of
MRSA infection and colonization; and they have the diagnosis of MRSA made in an outpatient setting or by culture
positive for MRSA within 48 hours after admission to a
hospital.[12]

CA-MRSA is resistant to fewer medications than HA-MRSA,
which makes it easier to treat than HA-MRSA. Less than 6 percent of all CA-MRSA cases become invasive. However, a new
strain of CA-MRSA secretes an especially dangerous toxin
known as Panton-Valentine leukocidin. If this strain gets into a
person's bloodstream, it can be deadly. It destroys soft tissue
and bone, and it causes a severe type of pneumonia that eats
away at the lungs. Author Jessica Snyder Sachs describes the
case of a woman stricken with this strain of CA-MRSA: "The in-
take nurse noticed shortness of breath, coughing, and hemop-

A new strain of community-acquired MRSA destroys soft tissue
and bone and causes a severe type of pneumonia, which eats away
at the lungs.

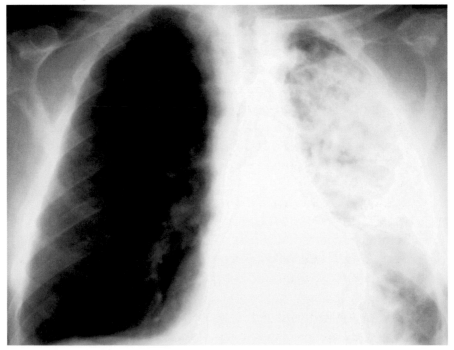

tysis, or blood-streaked sputum. . . . The woman was clearly suffering from bacterial pneumonia. . . . [By looking at a computed tomography scan of the patient's lungs, the doctor] could see gaping holes, some as large as an inch square, that riddled what should have been smooth lung tissue."[13]

Complicating Matters

Complicating matters, doctors are now diagnosing cases of CA-MRSA in hospitalized patients and cases of HA-MRSA in individuals who have not been in a health care facility. This is occurring because both types of the bacteria are becoming more common. As a result, increasing numbers of people are becoming colonized and/or infected, and these people are spreading the particular type of MRSA they carry. For instance, hospital patients and hospital visitors may enter the hospital already colonized with CA-MRSA and spread it to other patients. Conversely, formerly hospitalized individuals can easily spread HA-MRSA to the healthy people in which they come in contact. Bertha S. Ayi explains how this happens:

> How did people living in our communities going about their daily lives become infected with USA100 [a strain of HA-MRSA]? . . . They probably visited someone in the hospital or shared a bus ride or a personal item with someone with MRSA who had just left the hospital. Also we need to remember that all those who get MRSA in the hospital and are treated, ultimately go home. That person could be our grocery store sales person who packs our food with a smile, the sales person who hands you the movie tickets, the guy who just came in your home to fix your cable box or the lady who just handled your cell phone when it broke.[14]

People at Risk

Because MRSA spreads so easily, anyone can contract it. Certain people, however, are at greater risk. These include people who are colonized with MRSA and their family members; hospitalized individuals; individuals with compromised immune systems; individuals with indwelling medical devices such as artificial joints, catheters, and heart valves; illegal drug users; individuals with occupational exposure, such as health care workers, police, and firefighters; contact sport athletes; and people living in crowded environments, such as prison inmates, college students, military personnel, and residents of homeless shelters.

CA-MRSA in Prison Populations

The rates of CA-MRSA among prison inmates, for example, are comparable to the rates of HA-MRSA in hospitalized patients. Between 1996 and 2002 the number of MRSA cases in Texas state prisons alone was 10,942, with three deaths. A 2006 study conducted by researchers at the University of Maryland, Baltimore, which looked at risk factors for MRSA, found that prisons are "focal points for transmission of emerging infections. . . . [Prisons are] epidemiological [contagious disease] engines that drive the unfolding MRSA epidemic."[15]

Prison inmates live in close quarters, often share contaminated items, may have poor hygiene, and have high rates of immunosuppression diseases, which make them more vulnerable. Similar conditions exist in homeless shelters, making the homeless vulnerable. Illegal drug users who share needles, crack pipes, and other drug paraphernalia that can carry MRSA are also in harm's way. Law enforcement officers and firefighters are routinely exposed to these high-risk groups, which puts them at risk, too. In 2006, for example, fifteen law enforcement officers contracted MRSA while working in jails in Greenville, South Carolina.

Infections in Athletes and Gym Members

Athletes, especially those who participate in contact sports like football, basketball, soccer, and wrestling, are also vulnerable. These athletes come in close contact with each other. Artificial turf, wrestling mats, gym equipment, and towels can harbor MRSA. Because athletes routinely get cuts and scrapes, the bacteria have easy access into their bodies. Boone Baker, who played wide receiver for Austin High School in Texas, contracted a life-threatening MRSA infection in 2005 when his left shoulder crashed into the artificial turf. According to Robert Daum, head of infectious diseases at the University of Chicago Children's Hospital, "A lot of athletes are playing with cuts in their skin. Or on Astroturf, which is like a rug and can burn, abrade your skin. Staph love it when we have a break in our skin. They love it. They say, 'This is just what I need to get inside.'"[16]

All levels of athletes are at risk. Fifty-three percent of 364 high school and college athletic trainers surveyed in 2006 reported having treated MRSA in athletes in their care. As Ron Courson, the director of sports medicine at the University of

Bacteria or Virus?

Bacteria and viruses both cause infections, but the two are quite different. Bacteria are ten to one hundred times larger than viruses. Some bacteria are beneficial, whereas viruses have almost no beneficial function.

A virus's only purpose is to replicate. It cannot do so on its own. Viruses must get inside a living cell in order to multiply. Because they cannot replicate on their own, viruses are not considered truly living creatures. Bacteria, on the other hand, are independent living microorganisms. They can grow and multiply on almost any surface.

Bacteria and viruses attack the body differently. Bacteria secrete toxins that harm the body. Viruses use material in body cells to replicate. One virus can turn into 1 million in a matter of hours. Newly formed viruses burst out of the host cells, destroying the cells in the process. They then move on to other cells.

Because bacteria are alive, they can be killed. Antibiotics are chemicals that destroy bacteria. Because viruses are not technically alive, antibiotics cannot destroy them. Treatment of most viral infections involves relieving the symptoms rather than destroying the virus.

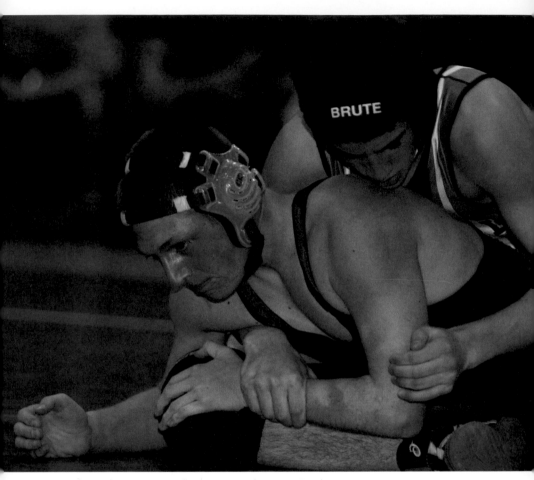

MRSA bacteria can live on towels, mats, and sports equipment, making athletes more vulnerable to MRSA—especially if they have an open scrape or cut.

Georgia, explains, "You'd be hard pressed to find an athletic setting—whether high school, intercollegiate or professional—that has not been exposed to MRSA."[17]

For example, a Texas study reported that 276 high school football players were infected with MRSA between 2003 and 2005. The University of Southern California reported thirteen cases of MRSA in its football team in 2002 and six cases in 2003. Complications from the illness caused the deaths of University of Tulsa football player Devin Adair in 2006 and Pennsylvania's Lycoming College football player Ricky Lannetti in 2003.

Professional athletes are also susceptible. Since 2003, the Washington Redskins, the St. Louis Rams, the San Francisco 49ers, the Pittsburgh Steelers, the Miami Dolphins, and the Cleveland Browns football teams have reported cases of MRSA. Professional basketball and baseball teams also have been dealing with the condition. In 2005 baseball player Sammy Sousa contracted a MRSA infection from contaminated carpet in the team's locker room.

It is clear that MRSA spreads easily. Although certain factors increase an individual's risk of contracting the condition, no one is safe. And, because bacteria keep changing in order to survive, emerging strains of MRSA are proving to be ever more dangerous. Once the bacteria get into the bloodstream, the results can be lethal. Seeking prompt treatment helps keep individuals safe.

CHAPTER TWO

Symptoms, Diagnosis, and Treatment

MRSA infections can become life threatening if they enter the bloodstream. The infection can progress from a minor skin infection to a potentially deadly condition in a few days. Prompt treatment helps prevent this from happening. However, because symptoms vary depending on where the infection has taken hold and its severity, diagnosing the condition is difficult. The severity and location of the infection also impacts the treatment, which varies accordingly.

It Might Look Like a Spider Bite

A MRSA infection can cause a wide range of symptoms. The infection usually first appears as a boil, or a pimplelike bump that looks like a spider bite. In reaction to the infection, the immune system sends blood filled with disease-fighting white blood cells to the area. This causes the infected area also to become red, swollen, warm, and painful, all characteristics of inflammation, which is the body's way to combat dangerous microorganisms. Pus, another characteristic of inflammation, fills the boil or "spider bite," turning it into an abscess.

Left untreated, the infection is likely to invade and destroy surrounding tissue. In response, the immune system signals the brain to set the body's temperature higher, producing fever

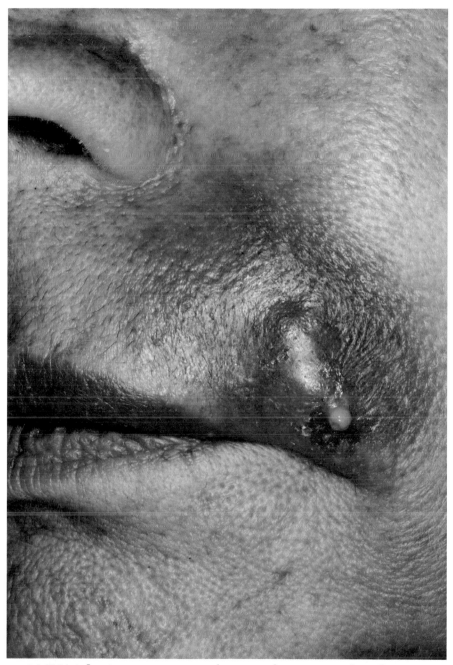

A MRSA infection can cause a wide range of symptoms. The infection usually first appears as a boil, or a pimplelike bump that looks like a spider bite.

and fatigue. This, too, is a sign of inflammation and is done as a defense against bacteria, which thrive at normal body temperature but weaken if the temperature rises. Bertha S. Ayi describes the symptoms of one of her patients, named Tom:

> One morning he noticed a small red bump on his thigh, which he thought was a spider bite. The bump became swollen, and by the next day it burst open releasing blood and other fluid. The area around the bump up to Tom's groin became hot, red, and painful. Within the next few days Tom's knee became swollen and infected and he developed a high fever. At this point, he was admitted to the hospital with a diagnosis of MRSA.[18]

No Body Part Is Safe

Left untreated, the infection can get into the bloodstream in a matter of days. If this occurs, other, more serious symptoms arise. For instance, some strains of MRSA produce toxins that destroy bones. When high school football player C.J. Jackson was infected with MRSA, the infection got into the bones in his knee, toes, and hip. "It was eating my bones from the inside out,"[19] he explains.

Some strains release toxins that cause a deadly form of pneumonia, which can kill a person in just a few hours. Still other toxins can cause dangerous blood clots. If a blood clot lodges in an artery or vein, blood flow may be inhibited. This can lead to heart attacks or strokes. In the lungs, a blood clot can make breathing difficult. If blood flow to the hands or feet is compromised, healthy cells in the fingers, toes, hands, and feet can become gangrenous, which means they die and begin to decompose. Left untreated, gangrene spreads and can be fatal. Often, the only way to save the patient is to amputate the infected part. Green Bay, Wisconsin, teenager DaVonte King had his left leg amputated in 2007 after contracting an invasive MRSA infection while playing football.

If the bacteria attack a vital organ, the bacteria and the toxins they secrete can compromise that organ's ability to function or cause it to fail. If MRSA infects the brain, it can cause meningitis, a dangerous disease. If it infects the heart, it can cause a condition called endocarditis, an infection of the inner lining of the heart and/or the heart valves, which can be fatal.

No body part is safe. MRSA can infect the spine, causing paralysis. It can spread into the eyes or ears, causing blindness and/or deafness. It can cause the liver and kidneys to cease functioning. The case of sixteen-year-old MRSA survivor Boone Baker is a prime example. The infection attacked his spine, spread into his right eye, and caused a blood clot to form in his lungs.

Michelle, another MRSA survivor who contracted the infection after surgery, had a similar experience. She explains:

> The MRSA developed on the wound. Approximately 7 days after the surgery I was diagnosed. I remained in the hospital for about a month and still in a very ill condition was discharged to a skilled nursing home facility. I was too ill to remain there and was sent to another hospital where I was immediately diagnosed with sepsis [bacteria in the bloodstream], acute kidney failure, heart, liver and lung malfunctions. . . . This all happened when the MRSA became a systemic infection causing organ shutdown. Today I have permanent damage to my heart, kidneys and lungs.[20]

When the Body Overreacts to Infection

The body's reaction to the spreading infection causes still other problems. Because the presence of MRSA is so dangerous in the bloodstream and vital organs, the immune system often overreacts in an attempt to fight the infection. Fever can rise dangerously, climbing as high as 107 degrees Fahrenheit (42°C). Such high fevers can lead to a rapid pulse and breathing rate as well as severe dehydration, which can cause excess thirst, an inability to urinate, extreme fatigue, and mental confusion.

At the same time, small blood vessels known as capillaries widen so that blood can be rushed to the part of the body that harbors the infection. This leaves less blood in the center of the body for the heart to pump to other organs. As a result, blood pressure drops and the heart can pump only slowly and

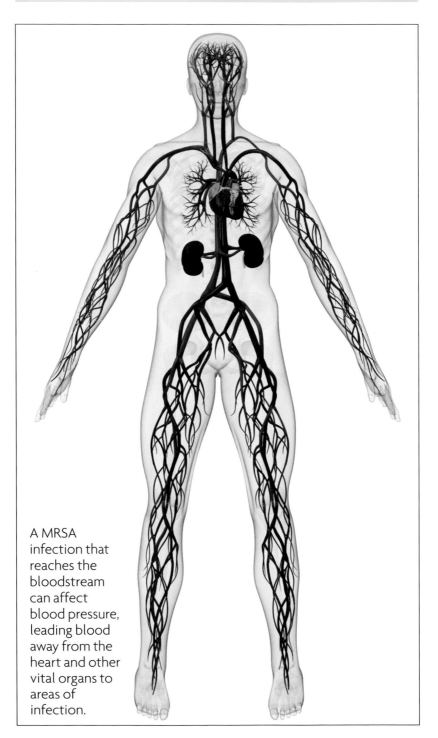

A MRSA infection that reaches the bloodstream can affect blood pressure, leading blood away from the heart and other vital organs to areas of infection.

with less force than it usually does. Therefore, less blood is pumped to the body, and the vital organs do not get the oxygen and nutrients they need to function. If normal blood pressure is not reestablished, the body goes into shock, which can cause multiple organ failure and death.

Diagnosing MRSA

Because MRSA can have so many different symptoms, diagnosing the condition is tricky. This is especially true in CA-MRSA because health care professionals are less likely to consider an infection in otherwise healthy individuals. It is common for early-stage infections to be confused with a spider bite, poison ivy, the flu, or a common staph infection. Marshall Jones, who was hospitalized for thirty-three days due to a MRSA infection, was originally diagnosed with a spider bite. His wife explains:

> Sometime during the third week of August 2004, I was giving my husband, Marshall, his usual monthly haircut, and a day later an ingrown hair appeared on the back of his neck. I plucked the hair out with tweezers and went on with our day. His wound continued to get worse that day, and the next, and he went to the doctor several days later to get it looked at, as the infection had turned into a large boil. Our doctor diagnosed it as a spider bite.[21]

Because time is of the essence in preventing the infection from entering the bloodstream, such misdiagnoses are dangerous. As Robert Daum explains, "We've seen lots of kids that come in here that needed intensive care and in fact have died that started off by being out in the community, where they get an . . . [inappropriate] treatment and then come in here having failed it."[22]

Culturing and Identifying Bacteria

The only way to accurately determine that the problem is, indeed, MRSA is to take a sample of infected skin cells, pus, urine, sputum, and/or blood. Samples can also be taken from indwelling medical devices such as catheters. The sample is then sent to a laboratory, where it is cultured. This means the sample is placed in a dish of nutrients, which encourages bacterial growth. If bacteria grow, the results are positive; if not, the results are negative.

Trained specialists examine the culture under a microscope. Once they establish the presence of bacteria, they then determine the particular type. Different germs or pathogens can be identified by their shape, size, and the way they move. *S. aureus* bacteria are yellow and resemble a cluster of grapes. Once it is determined that the bacteria are *S. aureus*, the bacteria are treated with different antibiotics, including methicillin, to establish if there is resistance to them. If the bacteria are not susceptible to methicillin, it is identified as MRSA. This procedure also helps the doctor to learn which antibiotics are most effective in treating the infection.

Other Diagnosing Tools

Although culturing the bacteria is the most accurate way of diagnosing MRSA, it is slow. It takes one to two days for a MRSA culture to grow. In cases of serious MRSA infections, rapid treatment is essential. In 2008 the U.S. Food and Drug Administration approved the use of a blood test that detects a gene sequence unique to MRSA in only about two hours. The test requires an expensive instrument that is not commonly found in most health care facilities. And, it is not as accurate as culturing the bacteria. It is, therefore, not as popular as the traditional test. However, it can provide a tentative diagnosis when time is of the essence.

In addition, a computed tomography (CT) scan may be administered. During a CT scan, patients lie on a moving table that passes through an imaging machine. Like an X-ray, it takes pictures of the body. But instead of taking pictures of bone, it takes pictures of soft tissue. Examining these pictures helps doctors to determine how deeply the infection has spread.

The First Steps for Treatment

Once a diagnosis is made, treatment begins. The goal of MRSA treatment is to clear the bacteria from the body. This is done in a

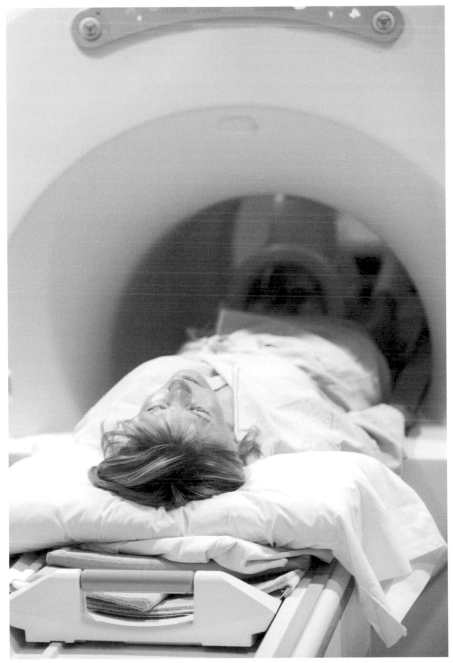

During a CAT scan, the patient lies still on a table while the imaging machine takes scans of the patient's soft tissue, where the infection may be found.

number of ways. The first step is to open and drain the abscess. Sometimes people try to do this themselves, but this is not wise. Squeezing or poking a skin infection can push the bacteria further into the body, worsening the infection, which is why this procedure should be left to a health care professional.

First, the health care professional makes an incision above the abscess. Next, he or she carefully drains out pus and other infected fluids. In some cases, more than 1 ounce (28.35g) of fluid may be drained. Depending on the severity and size of the abscess, this procedure may be done in a doctor's office with the use of a local anesthetic, which simply numbs the area to

Understanding the Cause of Infectious Disease

Until the 1860s, the cause of infectious diseases was unknown. Most physicians thought that mysterious substances that spontaneously developed inside a person's body caused infectious diseases. French scientist Louis Pasteur came up with another theory. He was studying what caused milk to sour. He found that the cause was bacteria. He theorized that if bacteria caused milk to go bad or sour, it could also cause problems in the body, which would result in infectious disease. He then tried to determine the origin of bacteria. Through other experiments, he discovered that bacteria come from the environment. He theorized, therefore, that bacteria get into the body from the outside in. This became known as the germ theory of disease.

Based on Pasteur's research, German scientist Robert Koch began looking at specific infectious diseases. As a result, between 1870 and 1883 he isolated the bacteria that cause anthrax, tuberculosis, and cholera. Koch's work helped to prove the germ theory was correct. Soon other scientists were looking at the causes of different infectious diseases. As a result, in 1899 Dutch scientist Martinus Beijerinck discovered viruses.

be incised. If the case is more serious, it is done in a hospital by a surgeon.

Debriding the Wound

Once the fluid is cleaned out, the doctor cuts away any dead or damaged tissue in or around the infected area in a procedure known as debridement. This helps eliminate, or at least reduce, bacterial colonies. Moreover, by removing dead and damaged tissue that has been stimulating inflammation, the procedure lessens the inflammatory process.

Small wounds can be debrided in a doctor's office. Larger wounds require surgery in a hospital setting. In one such surgical example, a woman had a MRSA infection that damaged tissue in her ankle. She describes her experience: "The surgery I had was wound debridement. They basically went in there and took all the tissue infected with MRSA out of my ankle/foot, so I would heal faster. Sometimes this can be done without surgery. . . . In my case . . . they had to surgically go in there and do it this way."[23]

After the sore is drained and debrided, it is cleaned with an antiseptic. Wounds are left to heal from the inside out. They are not stitched closed. This ensures that if any remaining bacteria or other pathogens get into the wound, they will not be sealed inside the warm, dark environment in which bacteria thrive. So, instead of closing the wound, it is packed with surgical dressing treated with an antiseptic that must be changed frequently.

Applying a Wound Vac

In cases in which the infection is severe and pus keeps building up even after the wound has been drained, a device known as a wound vac is applied to the wound. It applies constant suction to the wound, which removes pus and other fluids that harbor bacteria and stimulates new tissue to grow. A CA-MRSA survivor describes his experience:

> I had gotten poison ivy, which was almost gone. I had a small scabby part left on my foot and next to it a small

pimple was forming. Well, that little pimple on my foot had gotten worse. . . . Much worse—like I had elephantitis of the foot. . . . [I saw] a local surgeon the next day. I came, a doctor came in, looked at my foot and left within seconds without saying a word and came back with another surgeon. He said, "That must hurt A LOT." They made arrangements for me to go to a hospital. . . . I arrived at the hospital on Wednesday and had my first surgery the next day to open and clean . . . my foot. Wound vacs were on my foot at this point for the next two weeks, one week with a portable vac at home.[24]

Prescribing Powerful Antibiotics

The next step in treatment is the administration of antibiotics. Even when an abscess appears to be completely drained and cleaned, there is still a possibility that some bacteria were left behind. Therefore, patients are also prescribed antibiotics as part of treatment. Bertha S. Ayi explains:

> I have had patients ask me about the need for antibiotics if a boil has already been opened up and drained. I have likened an infection to a house that suddenly got invaded by rats or a bunch of ants. One possible way to get rid of these pests is to manually capture them or just physically get rid of them. But there may be some hiding in corners of the house that can then multiply and repopulate the house again. Spraying the house with the right pesticide can get rid of the pests. Antibiotics act like the spray. They ensure that all vestiges of infection have been eradicated to reduce the chance of recurrence.[25]

The specific medication that is administered depends on the laboratory findings of the original bacterial culture. In most cases, there is at least one medication, vancomycin, and often others, to which the bacteria are susceptible. Patients may be given just one antibiotic or a combination.

In mild cases, antibiotics are administered in capsule or pill form. Patients are instructed to finish the full prescription and not stop when they feel better. This helps ensure that the

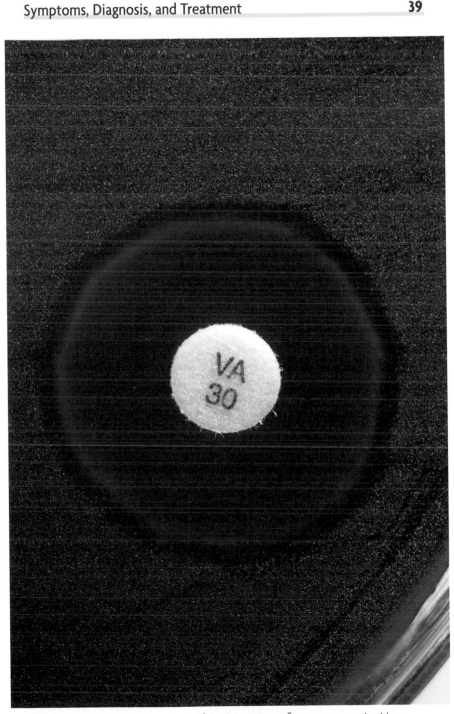

MRSA is resistant to most antibiotics except for vancomycin. Here, the bacteria did not grow around the white vancomycin tablet.

The Immune System

When an infection attacks the body, the immune system, which serves as the body's defense against diseases, fights back. Through a series of events known as an immune response, the immune system produces white blood cells, which attack foreign substances that gain entry into the body.

There are different types of white blood cells. Each has a specific job. Neutrophils are the most common white blood cell. They release chemicals that kill bacteria. Dead neutrophils release pus.

Basophils and eosinophils are less common. Eosinophils attack parasites. Basophils are involved in causing inflammation, characterized by fever, swelling, vomiting, and other symptoms, which help rid the body of germs.

Lymphocytes, which form cells known as T and B cells, attack both bacteria and viruses. B cells produce antibodies, or chemicals that lock onto and destroy specific pathogens. T cells detect and destroy viruses and bacteria. T cells also control inflammation because out-of-control inflammation can be dangerous.

toughest remaining bacteria are destroyed. In more serious cases, patients are admitted to the hospital, where antibiotics are administered intravenously. Administering medication intravenously gets the medication into the patient's bloodstream fast. Moreover, there is no oral form of certain extremely powerful antibiotics, such as vancomycin. Reality-television star Jack Mackenroth, who appeared on *Project Runway* in 2007, developed a MRSA infection in his mouth. He recalls:

> I was in the hospital for five days. I had to have an IV of really hardcore antibiotic—twice a day for five days. The good thing about this is if you catch it quickly enough, it goes away as quickly as it comes. It was weird, as soon as they give you the antibiotics, you kinda feel fine. I was kinda sitting in the hospital like, "Ugh, I'm bored."[26]

When MRSA Threatens Lives

When the infection has spread into the patient's bloodstream, additional treatment is required. At this point, MRSA is considered a medical emergency. If the patient has gone into shock, steps are taken to counteract the effects of shock. Such steps include administering fluids intravenously, which improves blood circulation and raises blood pressure. Providing oxygen through an oxygen mask is another important measure. It helps the patient to breathe more easily and increases the supply of oxygen to the bloodstream. At the same time, antibiotics

Some MRSA patients require lifesaving treatment, like kidney dialysis, if their organs are failing.

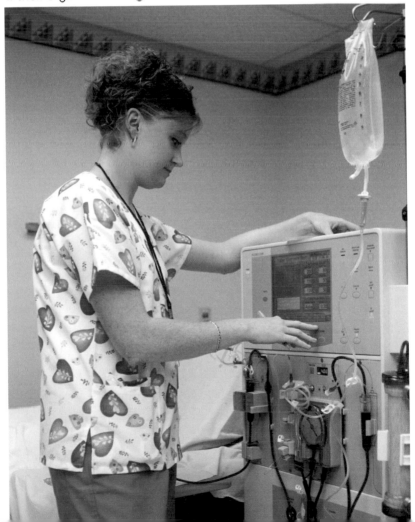

and other drugs are administered, including anti-inflammatory drugs, which lessen the effects of inflammation, and vasoconstrictors, which cause the capillaries to narrow and force pooled blood back to the heart.

Once patients are stabilized, they are admitted to the hospital's intensive care unit. Here, they are kept separate from other patients. Health care professionals don special gowns, masks, and gloves when they enter the room. This is done in order to keep the bacteria from being transmitted to others.

Otherwise, MRSA patients are treated just like other patients in the intensive care unit. They are attached to various machines that check how well their vital organs are functioning. These machines are connected to monitors in the patient's room and at the nurses' station. If the monitors indicate that organs are failing, special life-support machines assist compromised organs while patients heal.

For instance, if the infection has compromised the kidneys and the patient is unable to urinate, the patient will be attached to a dialysis machine. It is an artificial kidney that removes waste from the blood that would ordinarily be eliminated through urination. If the infection has caused pneumonia or has affected the patient's ability to breathe, the patient may be attached to a ventilator—a machine that breathes for the patient. Donna Wright, the mother of twelve-year-old MRSA survivor Hannah Ryan, describes her daughter's experience:

> Hannah's severe lung infection caused respiratory failure. . . . Because she could not breathe on her own, Hannah was put on an ECMO machine or Extracorporeal Membrane Oxygenation, a temporary support system that takes over for the lungs and heart. . . . Hannah also went into acute renal failure and she had to be put on a kidney support system. . . . Hannah was also fed through a tube in her stomach.[27]

In addition, in cases in which the infection cannot be well controlled, patients may require multiple surgeries to repeatedly clean, drain, and debride the infected areas. Ten-year-old Daniel Hunt, for example, had to undergo five operations when a MRSA infection got into his bones.

Fortunately, most cases of MRSA do not require multiple surgeries. Most do not spread into the bloodstream and threaten lives. But some infections do become serious. When individuals notice unusual skin infections, the best way to avoid a severe infection is to seek immediate medical attention. Mike Gansey, a MRSA survivor and former professional basketball player, puts it this way: "People have lost their lives from this, have lost body parts. It's something you don't want to mess around with, and if you see any little thing that looks suspicious, get it checked out. You never know what it could be."[28]

CHAPTER THREE

Living with MRSA

Living with a MRSA infection is challenging. Recovery from an infection can also be difficult. Some individuals face a prolonged recovery period. "I had missed work for a month and I'm now getting back," a thirty-seven-year-old MRSA survivor explains. "The physical and emotional toll it took on me and my family . . . was incredible."[29] And, because MRSA infections frequently recur, anyone who has been infected with MRSA is faced with the threat of becoming reinfected.

Taking steps to deal with these issues helps individuals to cope. Peg McQueary, whose recovery has lasted three years and has been peppered with recurring MRSA infections, explains: "I hope to just be able to have the strength to . . . do the things that we used to do before I got sick and just take it one day at a time. Deal with it one day at a time. If another boil comes, we deal with it. Just as we've been doing for the last three years."[30]

Prolonged Antibiotics Administration

Recovering from MRSA can be a slow process. To clear any trace of the bacteria from the body, most patients need to take antibiotics for anywhere from ten days to several months, depending on the severity of the infection.

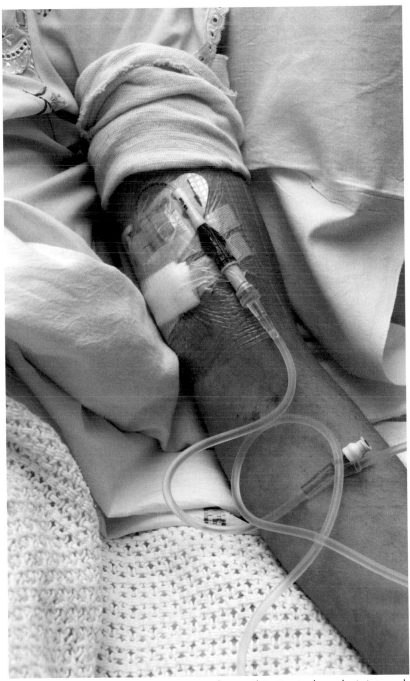

In severe cases, it is often necessary for antibiotics to be administered daily via a PICC line.

In severe cases, it is often necessary for the antibiotics to be administered intravenously. In these cases, patients may receive these treatments at home with help from a visiting nurse, as an outpatient in a hospital, or as a patient in a long-term care facility such as a nursing home. Teenager C.J. Jackson, for example, spent eleven days in the hospital due to a severe MRSA infection. When he was released from the hospital, he was put on intravenous antibiotic treatment at home for a month. Then, he took antibiotics orally for nine months.

Receiving daily doses of intravenous medication is not pleasant. Patients have to endure repeated needle sticks or be tethered to the intravenous pole, which limits their mobility. To meet this challenge, many individuals with MRSA are fitted with a peripherally inserted central catheteter (PICC). It is a long, thin, flexible tube that is inserted into a vein, usually near the elbow. The tube is then threaded up the vein until the tip sits in a large vein above the heart. A drip line is attached to the outside end of the tube. Intravenous medication is administered through this drip line. A bandage is placed over the insertion site, which keeps the PICC line in place. This allows patients to live a more normal life during their recovery. They can move around without worrying about the PICC line coming loose, and they do not have to suffer from frequent needle sticks.

Although a PICC line offers many benefits, it also presents several problems as an indwelling device. Bacteria can colonize the tubing and enter the body through the insertion point. This puts patients at risk of becoming reinfected with MRSA or contracting another type of bacterial infection. Making sure to keep the area around the insertion point clean helps individuals to avoid infection and cope with this challenge. Because MRSA can be carried on unwashed hands, it is essential that individuals wash their hands before and after handling the PICC line. It is also important to have the line changed at least every thirty days, which lessens the threat of a secondary infection developing.

The prolonged use of antibiotics, whether oral or intravenous, presents still more challenges. Antibiotics attack all bacteria in the body, including helpful bacteria. The loss of helpful bacteria gives harmful bacteria more space to colonize and stimulates the emergence of more powerful bacteria. Making matters worse, the antibiotics used to treat MRSA can cause unpleasant side effects. These include an upset stomach, dizziness, and fatigue.

Coping with Long-Term Treatment

Individuals cope with these problems in a variety of ways. One way is to take special medication designed to counteract the unpleasant side effects. Eating foods that are gentle on the stomach also helps to lessen stomach problems. And, because chemicals in certain foods may lessen the strength of some antibiotics, individuals often restrict such foods from their diet. Eating yogurt or drinking buttermilk—both of which contain helpful bacteria—is another way individuals keep harmful bacteria under control. These products put helpful bacteria back into a person's body.

Regular visits to a health care provider also help individuals to cope. Frequent blood tests track how well antibiotics are working and can identify the presence of a secondary infection before it causes major problems. Denise Rauff, whose daughter, Emily, had a MRSA infection, explains: "The medications that are effective against MRSA are powerful and they come with their own set of risks. Emily's blood count had to be monitored while on Zyvox [an antibiotic] and she had certain food restrictions."[31]

Wound Care

Another challenge that recovering individuals face is caring for open wounds. An abscess that has been opened, cleaned, and drained is usually packed with special dressing. To prevent infection and to allow the wound to heal properly, the dressing must be changed often. To meet this challenge, some individuals depend on a family member who has been trained to change the dressing. Others make frequent trips to the doctor. John, who had an infection in his chest, recalls:

> The doctor left the wound open because he said that sewing it closed would allow any bacteria still in there to

grow. It was a big hole, about the size of a half dollar in my chest, and pretty deep. He packed it with special gauze. For the first week, I had to go back to his office every day, so he could change the dressing. He used a tool that looked like a tweezer to pull the dressing out, and it came out in a long ribbon. Then he'd put new dressing back in. He really packed it in. It hurt when he did it, not intensely but it stung some. The next few weeks, I went every other day, then every few days, and eventually once a week. As the wound healed, the ribbon got shorter. Eventually, the flesh healed and the hole covered over. That's what healthy skin does. But it took a couple of months. The whole thing was stressful; it took up a lot of time going back and forth to the doctor. Also, there was always the chance that the wound would get re-infected, and then I would have had to go to the hospital for a larger surgery. But all in all, I didn't mind the whole thing. I did what I had to do to get better. I feel pretty lucky.[32]

A Weakened Body

More challenges arise after a severe MRSA attack, which can have an overwhelming effect on an individual's body. It is not uncommon for recovering patients to suffer from profound fatigue and weakness, above and beyond that caused by antibiotics. As MRSA survivor Tony Field recalls, "Lethargy was a problem. I could sit and doze in a half conscious and listless world for hours. . . . I would force myself to do things and convince myself that I was OK but I became tired so quickly it was painful."[33]

There are a number of steps that individuals take to manage their fatigue. Cutting back on daily activities is one step. This includes taking a leave of absence from work or school as well as turning to friends, family members, or professionals for help with routine tasks like cooking, housecleaning, driving, and shopping. Taking frequent naps is another way to combat fatigue. It helps people conserve energy and promotes healing. Michelle Wells, who was infected with MRSA along with her husband, daughter, and mother-in-law, advises, "Get LOTS of rest. . . . If you think and feel you need a nap and have a chance

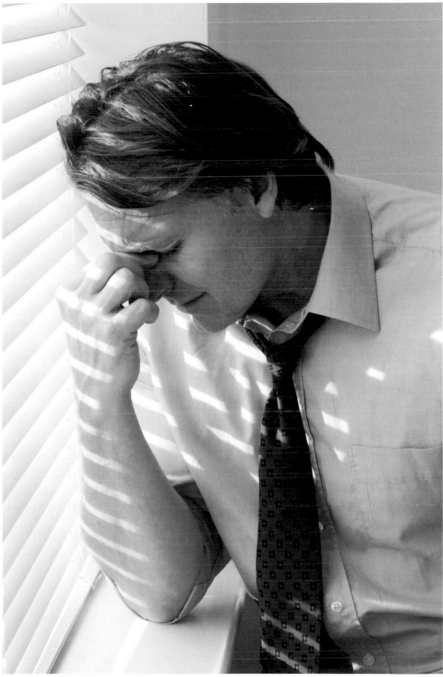

Even after recovery, MRSA leaves the body weak and fatigued. Some people have a hard time returning to their normal lives.

to do it, forget the mess in the kitchen it will be there when you wake up. People with MRSA get tired very easily and we need extra rest. Don't feel guilty for doing it."[34]

Pain is also a frequent problem. Tenderness and soreness are common after surgery. Weak and damaged tissue, muscle, and bones can be painful, too. "Since the infection, I've been battling severe fatigue and on-going problems with my leg and hip," explains Peg McQueary. "I only get 4–5 hours a day on my leg before it starts killing me. I have a constant limp, it swells and the pain in my hip and leg is unlike anything I've ever had."[35] Taking pain medication helps individuals to face this challenge. Such medication may be administered in pill form or as a patch that delivers the medication through the skin.

Participating in enjoyable activities that distract individuals from painful sensations is another way that patients deal with pain. Activities such as reading, watching a favorite television show or movie, playing a video game, listening to music, or visiting with family and friends are just a few activities that can help take a person's mind off pain.

Pets and MRSA

Dogs and cats can get MRSA. Just like humans, they can have active infections or be colonized and carry the bacteria. Humans can infect their pets, and pets can infect humans.

Experts advise people who get repeated MRSA infections to have their pets checked for the condition. Pets with MRSA are treated in the same manner as humans. Infected abscesses are cleaned and drained, and pets are administered antibiotics.

If a pet has MRSA, family members need to be careful not to touch the animal's infection, to use gloves while changing the pet's bandages, and to wash their hands after touching the pet. Infected pets should be kept off beds and furniture. Conversely, if a family member has MRSA, the pet should be kept away from infected wounds or contaminated bandages.

The Loss of Mobility

Another challenge is the loss of mobility. Individuals who have been bedridden for a long time, as well as those who have had a bone infection in a foot or leg, often have problems walking. Physical therapy helps these individuals to strengthen their muscles and regain their mobility. Often, patients who have weathered the severest MRSA attacks begin physical therapy while still in the hospital. Physical therapists use specialized equipment to assist patients to put weight on weakened legs. Once this is accomplished, patients are also taught to use adaptive equipment, such as a walker.

Upon their release from the hospital, many patients continue physical therapy sessions in an outpatient facility that resembles a gym. Under the supervision of a physical therapist, individuals perform individually customized exercises on weight training machines, pulleys, and other equipment. These exercises are designed to strengthen their bodies and increase their mobility. Hernan R. Chang explains how physical therapy helped his patient, Jeanne, who was bedridden for almost a month due to MRSA: "The physical therapist worked with her on a daily basis. Initially, Jeanne was not able to walk much. In fact, she was not even able to stand up without having her legs give out. Little by little, she improved and gained the confidence to walk the ward floor several times a day, at first with a walker and then by herself."[36]

The Threat of Recurrence

Although weakness, pain, extreme fatigue, and the loss of mobility do not usually affect individuals recovering from a mild MRSA infection, the threat of recurrence does. An estimated 10 to 30 percent of all individuals who have ever been infected with the bacteria suffer a recurrence. According to Robert Daum, "Recurrence is one of our biggest concerns with MRSA—it's a major, major problem."[37]

Even when patients are fully recovered, it is possible for some bacteria to survive treatment. These bacteria are likely to form a colony in the patient's nostrils or on the skin. Such colonies are

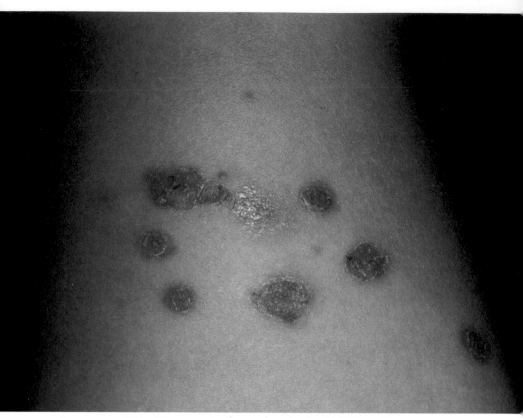

As many as 10 to 30 percent of people who had MRSA suffer a recurrence, sometimes in the form of impetigo or other skin rash.

usually too small to cause problems, but given the opportunity, the bacteria can reinfect the carrier, causing a recurrence.

Whereas some people do not suffer any recurrences, others have repeated infections and, therefore, must undergo frequent surgeries in which their wounds are opened, drained, and debrided. Jonathan Zenilman estimates that 25 to 35 percent of outpatient visits to the Johns Hopkins infectious disease clinic are recurring staph infections, many of which are MRSA. "These people are miserable," he explains. "You get recurring boils that can be difficult to control."[38]

Experts do not know why some individuals are more prone to recurrences than others. Yet they do know that recurrences are most likely to occur in patients with weakened immune systems. For example, 41 percent of individuals with HIV/AIDS who have been infected with MRSA become reinfected.

Survivors of MRSA do not have to be seriously ill for their immune systems to be vulnerable. Their defenses are weakened by the infection, the surgery, and the prolonged use of antibiotics. Stress, lack of sleep, poor diet, and minor illnesses such as a cold or the flu make matters worse. MRSA survivor Boone Baker's initial bout with MRSA was a mild skin infection, which healed after the infected area was cleaned and drained and antibiotics were administered. Three months later Baker contracted the flu. While his immune system was weakened by the flu, he suffered a near fatal recurrence of MRSA. "I thought it was completely behind us,"[39] his mother admits.

Living with the threat of recurrence can be stressful for individuals. As one woman who survived a severe MRSA infection and several recurrences explains, "I was diagnosed with MRSA in 2005. . . . Since then I have been on IV vancomycin at home twice, and in the hospital once. . . . It is very scary as you never know when it will hit you again."[40]

Preventing Recurrences

Taking steps to lessen the threat of a recurrence helps. Because MRSA can get into the body through tiny openings in the skin, proper skin care is vital. Avoiding activities that can cause skin wounds helps prevent reinfection. Such measures include refraining from scratching or picking at itchy wounds, sores, or insect bites. Likewise, MRSA survivors should use electric razors rather than manual ones. This is because an electric razor is less likely to cause small nicks and cuts. Using creams and ointments to fight dry skin, which cracks easily, is another measure. Not getting tattoos or body piercings, not participating in contact sports, and wearing gloves while doing manual labor also protects the skin.

When cuts and scrapes do occur, disinfecting them as soon as possible and covering them with a bandage to help keep dirt and bacteria out is vital. Changing bandages frequently, rather than keeping them on for several days, also lessens the possibility of infection.

Decolonization, which is a process aimed at destroying MRSA colonies in individuals' nostrils and on their skin, is another step that helps some people. It involves putting a powerful antibiotic ointment into the nostrils three to four times a day, showering twice a day with an antiseptic solution, and taking an oral antibiotic over the course of a week.

Because some health experts are concerned that MRSA may develop resistance to the antibiotic ointment administered during decolonization, the process is somewhat controversial. Decolonization is used most often only in people who suffer from frequent infections.

Also, MRSA colonies often re-form when decolonization treatment ends. About 50 percent of individuals become recolonized within a year; conversely, 50 percent do not. Writer Erin Zammett Ruddy and her infant son, Alex, are plagued with frequent MRSA infections. She is hoping decolonization will help them. Here is what she has to say about it:

> We . . . [are] still dealing with MRSA, the lovely staph infection Alex and I picked up in the hospital where I gave birth. . . . We were recently advised to do a "decolonization." Alex had his third "breakout," which is really just an ugly looking sore in his diaper area, but still scary. . . . Well, it's been a while, but we're finally ready to kill this thing once and for all. So beginning this weekend we will be bathing in Hibiclens [an antiseptic skin cleanser], shoving Bactraban [an antibiotic ointment] up our noses three times a day and dousing our hands with Purell [hand sanitizing gel] constantly. . . . I just pray we can get this thing put behind us but only time will tell. The doc said if six months go by without a breakout, there's a good chance we're MRSA free. Then after a year with no break outs we're in the clear.[41]

Strengthening the Immune System

Another way to lessen the chance of recurrence is to strengthen one's immune system. Getting eight hours of sleep each night and eating a healthy diet are steps that MRSA survivors take to boost their body's natural defenses. As an extra

Herbal Remedies and the Immune System

Some individuals try to strengthen their immune system with herbal remedies. Herbs are medicinal plants whose leaves, stems, seeds, and/or roots are believed to have healing properties. There is no conclusive evidence that herbs are effective, but many individuals believe that certain herbs stimulate the immune system, thereby helping them fight infection.

Echinacea, which is derived from coneflowers, is among these herbs. Herbalists say that it contains antibacterial properties and chemicals that stimulate the production of white blood cells.

Garlic also appears to have antibacterial properties. It has been used to ward off infection for centuries. During the thirteenth century, when the bubonic plague overwhelmed Europe, many individuals wore necklaces made from garlic in hopes of warding off the illness.

Ginseng is another herbal remedy. It appears to boost the body's defenses by strengthening the immune system and helping the body deal with stress.

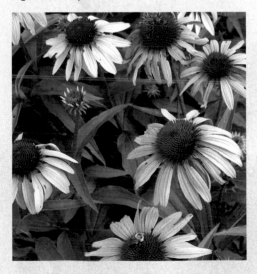

Herbalists say echinacea contains antibacterial properties and that chemicals in the plant stimulate the production of white blood cells.

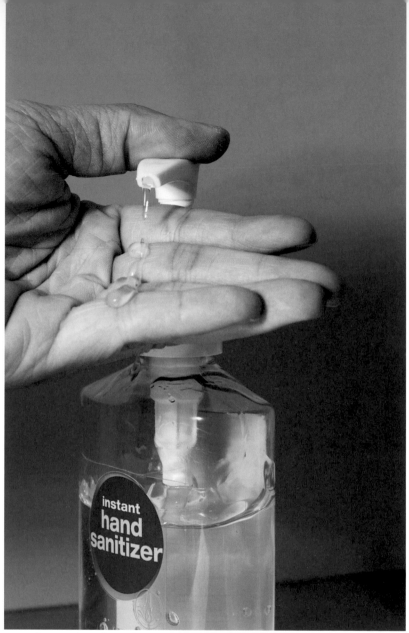

Disinfecting hands with sanitizer several times throughout the day can prevent the spread of germs and bacteria that might cause a MRSA recurrence.

precaution, some people supplement their diet with a multiple vitamin to ensure they are getting all the nutrients their immune system needs to function efficiently. Some also take a daily garlic capsule or add more garlic to their diets. Garlic is believed to have antibacterial qualities and may help fight infection. "Eat healthy," Michelle Wells advises. "Take vitamins if you can, it depends on the meds you are on if you can take vitamins or not. Make sure to ask the doctor. . . . MRSA breaks down the immune system and keeping healthy is needed."[42]

Getting an annual flu shot is another vital step, as is living a healthy lifestyle. Avoiding activities like smoking and abusing alcohol or drugs, which depress the immune system, is an additional measure that individuals may take.

Stress, too, has an adverse effect on the body's defenses. It triggers changes in the immune system that inhibit the production of infection-fighting white blood cells. Therefore, it is important to avoid stressful situations whenever possible and to participate in stress-reducing activities. These activities include meditating and mind-body exercises like yoga and tai chi as well as relaxing hobbies such as playing an instrument, painting, and gardening, to name a few.

Getting exercise also boosts the immune system. Likewise, it improves sleep and lessens fatigue and stress. Although some recovering MRSA patients may not be able to participate in vigorous exercise at first, doing moderate exercise, such as taking a short walk or riding a bicycle, helps strengthen the body. And, as individuals get stronger, they can increase their level of exercise.

Jeanine Thomas, a MRSA survivor and the founder of the MRSA Survivor Network, an organization dedicated to raising MRSA awareness and preventing MRSA infections, does whatever she can to build up her immune system. She makes sure to get plenty of sleep, eats lots of fresh fruit and vegetables, and exercises often. She also avoids stressful situations and encounters with people who upset her. She also participates in volunteer activities, which she enjoys.

Living with MRSA can be difficult. A serious MRSA infection can take a tremendous toll on the body. Long-term antibiotic use also presents challenges. Likewise, no matter how minor the infection, there is always the threat of recurrence. When individuals take steps to strengthen and protect themselves, they make their recovery easier and reduce the possibility of the condition recurring.

CHAPTER FOUR

Preventing MRSA Infections

There is no way to completely prevent MRSA infections. There are, however, a number of measures that individuals can take to lessen the spread of the bacteria and protect themselves from becoming infected.

The Importance of Hand Washing

MRSA is spread through contact with the bacteria. Although it is not always possible to avoid such contact, commonsense health practices can provide protection. Hand washing is probably the most important way to stop the spread of infection and protect oneself. It loosens bacteria and washes it away. According to Chuck Kimmel, president of the Athletic Trainers' Association and head athletic trainer at Tennessee's Austin Peay State University, "If there was only one tool in the toolbox to fight MRSA, hand washing would be the most valuable one. The occurrence of MRSA would be significantly reduced if everyone washed their hands aggressively and often."[43]

Medical experts advise individuals to wash their hands before eating, drinking, or preparing food; before and after blowing their nose, touching sores, or changing bandages; and after using the bathroom, having contact with a sick person, or touching surfaces handled by many people, such as those in crowded public places. Health writer Bronwyn Harris explains:

> Without being obsessive, if there is a chance that your hands are dirty, or that you've touched something that sick people have touched, wash your hands! It will help prevent MRSA. Use an alcohol based gel if you cannot wash your hands. . . . If you can't get to water and soap it's a good idea to have hand sanitizer with you. Take precautions in public bathrooms. Since you don't know if other people have washed their hands before touching the door knobs and the water faucets, it's better to use a paper towel or tissue if possible to avoid touching these surfaces and prevent MRSA.[44]

MRSA infections can be greatly reduced if people remain diligent about washing their hands before eating and preparing food, and after using the bathroom.

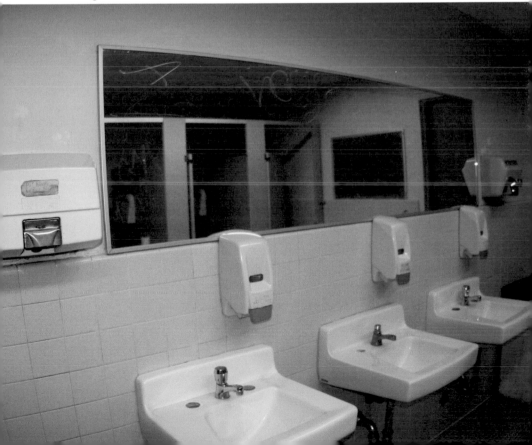

Hand-Washing Tips

To be most effective, hand washing must be done properly. This means washing with warm water and soap for at least fifteen seconds. Medical experts at the Mayo Clinic offer the following directions:

> Wet your hands with warm, running water and apply liquid or clean bar soap. Lather well. Rub your hands vigorously together for at least 15 seconds. Scrub all surfaces, including the back of your hands, wrists, between your fingers and under your fingernails. Rinse well. Dry your hands with a clean or disposable towel. Use a towel to turn off the faucet.[45]

In order to know how long to scrub, individuals are advised to recite the alphabet or sing the "Twinkle, Twinkle, Little Star" song, both of which last about fifteen seconds. And, because MRSA can live on bar soap, medical experts warn that it is best to use liquid soap or a fresh bar of soap.

When soap and water are not available, an alcohol-based sanitizer, which contains at least 60 percent alcohol, is a good substitute. Individuals should apply about one-half teaspoon of the sanitizer to their hands, then rub their hands together until the product dries. Sanitizers kill MRSA within fifteen seconds after the hands are rubbed together.

Covering Wounds

Other important hygienic practices include cleaning and covering open sores, which serves two purposes. First, if the sore is not infected, it prevents the bacteria from entering the body. Second, if the sore is infected, it keeps the bacteria from contaminating others. If sores are leaking, putting extra dressing on them also helps keep the bacteria from infecting others. Wearing clothes that cover bandages or sores offers protection as well. Yet even if leaking sores are covered, it is best to avoid activities in which others can come in contact with the leakage, such as contact sports. Perspiration can cause bandages to loosen and bacteria to leak out.

MSRA and Children

People of any age can contract MRSA. Parents of young children can take steps to protect them. One step is keeping toddlers from licking or biting the handle of grocery carts, where MRSA can grow. Another step is to bring a child's own toys to doctor appointments rather than letting the child play with the toys provided in the waiting room. The toys in the waiting room have been handled by many children and can harbor MRSA. In addition, babies should not be allowed to crawl on the floor in waiting rooms or other public places. Carpets can contain MRSA.

School-age children can take other precautions, such as carrying antiseptic wipes with them. Students should use the wipes to clean their hands when soap and water is not available.

Teachers and school administrators can help, too. They can ensure that environmental surfaces such as desks, locker rooms, and cafeteria tables are kept clean. They can also require all students to shower after physical education class and wash hands before lunch.

It Is Not Always Good to Share

Because MRSA can easily be transferred to almost any surface, sharing personal items such as clothes, earrings, cosmetics, towels, razors, nail files, and bar soap, among other things, is dangerous. "Don't share roll-on deodorant," Michelle Wells advises. "It could pass from one arm to the next if you happen to have MRSA boils [or a colony] in your arm-pits."[46]

Individuals should also be aware of shared items in places like nail salons, beauty shops, and tattoo parlors. If nail clippers, scissors, or needles are not properly sanitized, they can spread MRSA. Health writer Leslie Laurence gives these tips about protecting oneself in nail salons:

All nondisposable metal instruments should be in disinfectant such as Barbicide. Don't trust instruments that are pulled out of a drawer. Safer still, bring your own manicure and pedicure implements, as well as a mat for the tub. Don't shave your legs for 24 hours before or after a pedicure because bacteria can enter through nicks in your skin. Make sure your cosmetologist washes her hands and has no sores on them. Don't allow her to cut your cuticles or use a razor or grater on your calluses. And, if you have acrylic nails, don't allow use of an electric drill, which can penetrate and might have cut the person before you. Or bring your own drill bits.[47]

Before getting a salon treatment, like a pedicure, one must be sure that all instruments were disinfected in a solution like Barbicide.

Precautions for Athletes

Athletes often come in close contact with each other, and MRSA can settle onto many surfaces in gyms and locker rooms. It is especially important that athletes take steps to protect themselves and others. "Even if you are in good health, every bodybuilder should be concerned about the recent outbreak of methicillin-resistant Staphylococcus aureus (MRSA)," reports *Muscle & Fitness* magazine writer Dwayne Jackson. "After all, you invariably use the same bench, free weights, and cable attachments as many other people at your local gym and sharing athletic equipment is known to be a major risk factor for contracting this bacteria. So you should learn about MRSA and how to protect yourself when you work out."[48]

In addition to covering wounds and not sharing personal items, there are a number of other measures that athletes can take to stop the spread of MRSA. Not sharing sports equipment is one way. This is fairly simple when it comes to equipment like football helmets or protective pads; however, it is harder not to share large equipment, such as weight machines, free weights, and benches. Fortunately, there are precautions athletes can take to protect themselves and others. Wiping down the equipment before and after use is essential. Many gyms provide antiseptic spray and paper towels for this purpose.

In gyms where these are not provided, athletes are advised to bring their own antiseptic wipes. Personal equipment, such as helmets and pads, also should be wiped clean after use, and they should be dried before putting them away. Bacteria thrive in warm, dark, damp places. Storing damp sports equipment in a locker or a gym bag is a perfect environment for MRSA to grow. Experts at Athletic Management, a Web site for high school and college athletic directors, explain:

> Athletic equipment is supposed to keep the wearer safe, but if it's not properly taken care of, it can create a serious health hazard. When sweaty pads and uniforms are thrown into a bag or locker, the result is a warm, dark, moist environment that's perfect for MRSA bacteria to

grow. . . . Make sure padding and other equipment is stored somewhere where it can dry out between use.[49]

Putting a barrier between the skin and shared exercise equipment is another protective step. This includes wearing long sleeves, long pants, and weight-lifting gloves. Using a washcloth to grasp equipment also keeps MRSA off the skin. So does putting a clean towel between the skin and equipment like benches, mats, and bicycle seats. It is important to always put the same side of the towel or washcloth on the equipment and to keep this side from touching the skin. Marking the side that touches the equipment with a dot or an X helps. In addition, athletes should not dry themselves off with the towel they used on the equipment. They should use a fresh, clean towel. Health writer Bobbi Miller advises, "Make sure to . . . wrap a towel around the bar for squats, bench press, and any other lift where the bar will touch your body and possibly transfer staph infection. . . . Wear gloves to prevent MRSA from entering through the open skin in your hands. Make sure to throw your gloves in the wash when you get home."[50]

Showering after working out is also essential. It washes off any bacteria that may have been picked up while exercising or playing sports. Since his bout with MRSA, high school football player C.J. Jackson makes a point of showering after every game and practice. He explains: "Good sports hygiene is the most important thing. It's important to always take a shower after playing."[51]

Wearing flip-flops or shower slippers in the locker room is another way to stop infections from spreading. In 2006 ABC News conducted a test to find out how much harmful bacteria is found in a typical health club in New York City. News staffers wiped down exercise equipment, gym and locker room floors, and other surfaces to get bacterial samples. The samples were cultured and analyzed by Phillip Tierno, a microbiologist at New York University Hospital. Harmful bacteria were found everywhere, with the largest amounts on the locker room and shower floors. According to Tierno, "Unfortunately, germs do survive on the shower, on walls, and on the floor. I found it

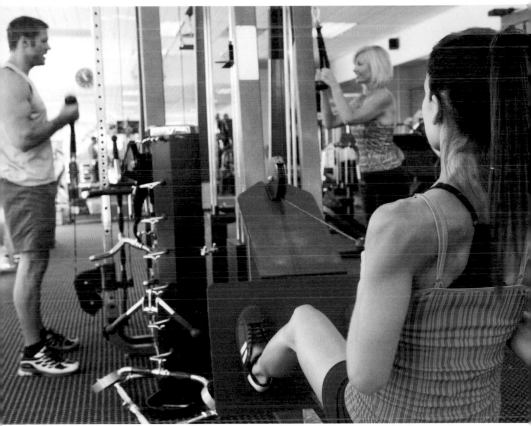

At the gym, it is important to wipe down all equipment before and after using it to avoid the spread of bacteria.

[harmful bacteria] in hordes—unbelievable quantities. . . . [But] you wear your little slippers, and you're OK."[52]

When a Roommate or Family Member Has MRSA

Individuals infected with or who carry MRSA and those who live with them take other precautions. By cleaning a shared shower after use with bleach or a cleanser with disinfectant, infected individuals help protect their loved ones. As Michelle Wells counsels, "Spray the shower with bleach and let it sit for about 15 minutes before you clean it. This needs to be done after each shower even when not broken out."[53]

Regular housecleaning also helps destroy MRSA. Because MRSA bacteria can live on most surfaces, it is vital to use a disinfectant daily to clean kitchen counters, faucets, doorknobs, light switches, refrigerator door handles, toilets, television remote controls, phones, pagers, and other frequently touched and shared surfaces. It is best to use a paper towel to wipe down these surfaces and then dispose of it. Wearing disposable gloves while cleaning and washing one's hands afterward also helps to keep the bacteria from being transferred to or from the cleaner's hands.

According to Washington State's Department of Health, individuals can use any cleaning product that has the word *disinfectant* on its label. Individuals can also make their own

Clothing and linens can harbor MRSA, and individuals with the infection must have their laundry washed seperately. Here, a hospital worker checks an inmate's identification before passing clean laundry through the door.

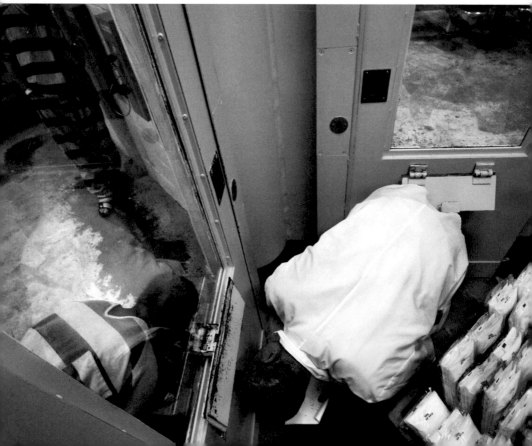

disinfectant by combining one tablespoon of bleach with a quart of water. Because bleach can evaporate, it is best to make a fresh mixture each time one cleans.

Clothing and linens can also harbor MRSA. Infected individuals should separate their laundry from that of other household members and wash their clothes and linens in hot water with a detergent that contains bleach. The laundry should then be dried in a clothes dryer. MRSA is not likely to survive the combination of the hot water, bleach, and dryer heat. If another member of the household handles an infected person's dirty clothes or linens, they should wear disposable gloves and wash their hands afterward.

Michelle Wells advises:

Wash everything in ALL hot water . . . then dry EVERY-THING to get that extra heat to kill the germs the wash didn't get. Bleach EVERYTHING! That goes for the darks as well the whites. They have color safe bleach now and works great. Bedding needs to be washed and or at least changed everyday when having an outbreak, at least 2 times a week when not having an outbreak. It's important. . . . Clean with bleach where ever and whenever you can. From the floors to the walls. . . . Use Lysol like [its] going out of style, spray down the phone, light switches, the key board and mouse, fridge door handles, door knobs, furniture, toilet, remotes, and so on. This needs to be done daily. . . . Wash the person who is infected, their clothes, towels, and wash cloths separate from others in the home. . . . Remember MRSA is all over the place. We don't want to add to the mess. So please be careful and thoughtful of others.[54]

Precautions at the Hospital

Because the majority of MRSA infections are hospital acquired, it is important that hospitalized individuals and their families take steps to protect themselves. According to Betsy McCaughey, the former lieutenant governor of New York and the founder of the Committee to Reduce Infection Deaths:

Staph germs race through hospitals because of unclean hands, contaminated equipment, bacteria-laden uniforms, and inattention to proper procedures. Amazingly, doctors fail to clean their hands before treating patients 52 percent of the time, according to research by infectious disease expert Didier Pittet, M.D. Equipment contaminated with bacteria—like stethoscopes—are used on one patient after another without being cleaned. Doctors and nurses carry bacteria from bedside to bedside on their lab coats and uniforms, and some hospital workers even wear their scrub suits out on the streets and then back to work.[55]

By insisting that hospital staff wash their hands before administering treatment, hospitalized individuals can reduce

Dangerous Clothing

Uniforms such as hospital scrubs and lab coats worn by health care professionals can be dangerous. They can easily pick up MRSA when health care workers lean over patients and brush against contaminated surfaces. To protect patients from MRSA, these clothes should be removed and laundered every day. Until about twenty years ago, most hospitals laundered uniforms for staff, but this is no longer the case. As a result, many health care professionals wear the same uniforms day after day. A 2009 University of Maryland study found that 65 percent of health care workers changed their lab coat less than once a week. Fifteen percent changed it once a month.

Wearing uniforms outside the health care facility spreads hospital-acquired MRSA to the community. For instance, when a health care worker sits down in a restaurant wearing infected scrubs, the bacteria can easily be passed to the table and chairs. The next person to sit down can then become infected.

Hospitals can help prevent the spread of MRSA by prohibiting hospital personnel from wearing scrubs and lab coats outside the building and by providing laundered uniforms for all staff members.

their risk of contracting MRSA. According to the Committee to
Reduce Infection Deaths:

> This is the single most important way to protect yourself
> in the hospital. If you're worried about being too aggres-
> sive, just remember your life could be at stake. All care-
> givers should clean their hands before treating you. . . .
> Don't be falsely assured by gloves. If caregivers have
> pulled on gloves without cleaning their hands first, the
> gloves are already contaminated before they touch you.[56]

Moreover, gloves should be discarded after a single use.

In addition, patients should ask their health care provider to
wipe down the flat surface of stethoscopes with alcohol before
using it on them. It can carry MRSA from patient to patient. Although the American Medical Association recommends physicians do this, few actually comply. It is also wise to ask that
blood pressure cuffs be placed over clothes because these, too,
can transfer MRSA to exposed skin.

Insisting that hospital visitors also wash their hands is another protective step. Having antiseptic wipes available helps
make this step easier. It is a good idea for patients to bring
wipes to the hospital with them, which they can offer visitors.

Protective Steps for Patients and Doctors

Patients can take other protective steps if they are having
surgery, such as asking potential surgeons their rate of infection for various procedures and selecting a physician accordingly. Showering with antibacterial soap and shampoo every
day for three to five days before having surgery is also a smart
move. This helps remove harmful bacteria from the skin before
it can cause an infection.

On the day of surgery, if body hair must be removed from the
surgical site, patients should ask that clippers be used rather
than a razor. Razors can cause small nicks through which
MRSA can get into the body. Making sure that antibiotics are
administered one hour before surgery also protects patients.
According to the American Healthcare Quality Association, doing so would avoid up to half of all surgical wound infections.

However, sometimes in the bustle before surgery, it is forgotten. "When the patient got down to pre-op, the pre-op nurse may have thought the nurse on the floor gave the antibiotic. So nobody really knew whether the antibiotic was given,"[57] explains Dale Braztler of the Oklahoma Foundation for Medical Quality. It is, therefore, important that patients remind health care providers when necessary. And because experts say that patients who are kept warm during surgery are less prone to developing infections, asking the doctor to take steps to keep the patient warm in the operating room makes sense. Requesting that the number of medical students and other nonessential personnel in the operating room be limited also helps. The more people present, the greater the risk of infection.

Other protective steps involve following proper procedures when introducing indwelling devices like central line catheters and urinary catheters. Because they break the skin, making it easy for bacteria to enter the body, and because MRSA can grow on the tubing, it is best to avoid indwelling devices whenever possible. If patients are alert and are able to use a bedpan, they do not need a urinary catheter.

When an indwelling device is necessary, patients should make sure that their skin is cleaned at the site of insertion. In addition, health care workers should always wear new gloves when inserting the catheter. Treating the catheter with antibiotics or an antiseptic also helps prevent infection. Likewise, because the longer that the line remains in place, the more time MRSA has to take hold, the catheter should be removed as soon as possible.

According to the Mayo Clinic, the threat of infection rises significantly when urinary catheters are left in place more than six days; intravenous lines should be changed every three days. CNN medical correspondent Elizabeth Cohen explains: "If you or a loved one has a urinary catheter in the hospital, be extra vigilant—they can become breeding grounds for bacteria. First, ask if one is truly necessary. . . . If you get one, make sure it comes out ASAP, since the longer it's in the riskier it becomes. Ask the same question about central line catheters, another potential host for bacteria."[58]

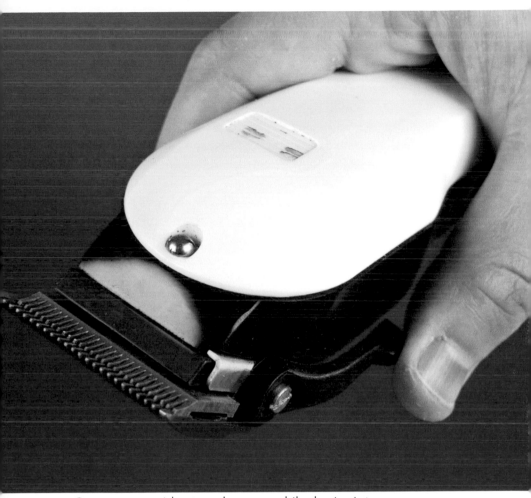

One way to avoid cuts and scrapes while shaving is to use an electric trimmer because the blades do not directly come into contact with the skin.

While recuperating, patients can take other protective measures. These include letting health care providers know if surgical dressings become loose or wet or if catheters loosen. Another protective measure is to always wear shoes or slippers when walking on hospital floors. Avoiding all contact with the wounds of other patients and not sharing books, newspapers, or other items also help keep MRSA from spreading. If the area around a hospital bed is dirty, patients should insist it be cleaned. Patients can also protect themselves by requesting that friends and family members who feel ill refrain from visiting.

Obviously, nobody wants to get a MRSA infection. Infected and colonized individuals, and health care providers, too, can take steps to protect others. Both healthy individuals and hospitalized patients can lessen their chance of contracting the illness by following simple health practices. "While the burden of decreasing the number of hospital infection cases lies with the health care system," explains award-winning medical journalist Peter Salgo, "patients can also take steps to protect themselves. Remember your mother was right: Wash your hands. . . . Being in charge of your health means being informed."[59]

CHAPTER FIVE

What the Future Holds

Infectious disease experts, scientists, health organizations, and government officials are working hard to reduce new cases of MRSA. Their primary focus is making hospitals safer. At the same time, some scientists are working on a vaccine against the bacteria. Others are investigating novel substances capable of destroying the bacteria.

Making Hospitals Safer by Screening Patients

Because the majority of MRSA infections are hospital acquired, health care organizations and professionals, government officials, and other interested parties are working hard to make hospitals safer. Achieving this goal involves a number of measures. One of the most important is screening incoming patients for MRSA, then taking precautions with patients who test positive in order to prevent them from transmitting the bacteria to others. These precautions involve isolating MRSA patients; having hospital personnel wear disposable gowns, masks, and gloves when treating MRSA patients; and keeping equipment used on MRSA patients away from other patients.

MRSA screening is not difficult or expensive. It involves taking a nasal or skin swabbing from every patient who is admitted

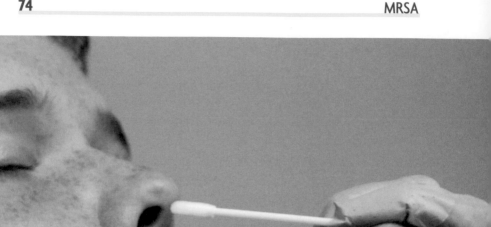

Incoming patients and hospital workers can be screened for MRSA with a nasal swab.

to the hospital. The swabbing is then cultured and examined for MRSA. Yet screenings are not commonly done. According to a 2007 survey by the Association of Professionals in Infection Control and Epidemiology, only about 29 percent of hospitals in the United States administer routine MRSA screenings. According to Betsy McCaughey:

Amazingly, most hospitals in the U.S. don't test incoming patients for MRSA.

Seventy to ninety percent of patients carrying MRSA are unknown. They are the silent reservoir in the hospital. Knowing which patient[s] are the sources of the bacteria is the key to stopping the spread. . . . Placing a patient in a room or even a wheelchair previously used by someone who unknowingly carried MRSA puts that patient at risk. When hospitals fail to identify which patients are carrying superbugs, hospital uniforms and equipment become conveyor belts for infection. When doctors and nurses lean over a patient with MRSA bacteria, their white coats and uniforms pick up that bacteria 65 percent of the time, allowing it to be carried to other patients.[60]

Those hospitals that have instituted MRSA screenings and take contact precautions with patients who test positive have shown a marked decrease in MRSA infections. For instance, the Department of Veterans Affairs cut MRSA infections by 50 percent in 150 of its hospitals; likewise, three Evanston, Illinois, hospitals reduced their infection rate by 60 percent. "The goal of the [MRSA screening] program was always to reduce the risk of MRSA infection to patients cared for," says Lance Peterson, an epidemiologist and the founder of the MRSA screening program in Evanston. "We want people to come here for health care and not go home with something unexpected that will later cause an infection."[61]

Other hospitals have been even more successful. The University of Pittsburgh Medical Center Presbyterian Hospital reduced MRSA infections by 90 percent, and the University of Virginia Hospital, which was plagued by MRSA outbreaks, virtually eliminated MRSA infections entirely. As Barry Farr of the University of Virginia Hospital explains, "Surveillance culturing—identifying every patient carrying the bacteria—was the key to thwarting the outbreak and eradicating MRSA."[62]

Because MRSA screening has proven so successful at reducing hospital-acquired MRSA infections, as of January 2009 three states—Illinois, New Jersey, and Pennsylvania—have passed

Poor Hygiene and Disease

During the seventeenth and eighteenth centuries, doctors and nurses rarely washed their hands or cleaned their instruments. As a result, infections were common. For instance, at that time, up to one-quarter of all women giving birth in Europe and America died of infection.

In 1847 Ignaz Semmelweis, a Hungarian physician, observed that infection rates dropped significantly when he insisted that medical students in his charge scrubbed their hands with powdered bleach between performing autopsies and delivering babies. He theorized that lack of proper hygiene spread infection. Semmelweis's peers dismissed his theory, which they considered insulting.

Over the next fifty years, other events proved Semmelweis's theory correct. For instance, English nurse Florence Nightingale found that infection rates dropped significantly among English soldiers when she scrubbed medical instruments and hospital ward floors and walls with powdered bleach.

British surgeon John Lister made a similar observance. He knew that fields in England, irrigated with raw sewage, were treated with carbolic acid to lessen unpleasant odors. He theorized that carbolic acid destroyed bacteria. So, he began cleaning surgical wounds with carbolic acid. He also made other surgeons in his hospital wash their hands and wear gloves.

laws requiring hospitals to screen all patients admitted to intensive care units for the bacteria. These patients generally have weakened immune systems, which put them at the greatest risk of contracting an invasive infection. Screening bills have also been introduced in California, the District of Columbia, Hawaii, Iowa, Kentucky, Maryland, Missouri, and Tennessee. Moreover, a bill sponsored by New Jersey senator Robert Menendez has been introduced to the U.S. Congress that would require hospitals to screen all patients for MRSA by 2012. As Lisa McGiffert, the director of the Consumers Union's

Stop Hospital Infections campaign, which supports the bill before Congress, explains:

> We know that MRSA infections are all too common in hos-
> pitals across the country, but most hospitals are not doing
> enough to protect patients. Screening patients for MRSA
> is a critical part of an effective strategy to stem the alarm-
> ing spread of these debilitating and sometimes deadly in-
> fections. . . . Stopping these infections from occurring in
> the first place is our best defense.[63]

Keeping Hospitals and Hospital Personnel Clean

Improving sanitary conditions in hospitals is another way to
make them safer. In an effort to save money, many hospitals
have trimmed their cleaning budgets. Groups dedicated to elim-
inating hospital-acquired infections, such as the Committee to
Reduce Infection Deaths, are working to pass legislation that
would require hospitals to make their infection rate public.

Being able to access such information, these groups say,
would help patients to make an educated choice when selecting a hospital. It is likely that patients would bypass hospitals
with high rates of infection. The threat of losing revenue would
encourage hospitals to spend more money on cleaning in order
to lower their infection rate.

Currently twenty-six states and the District of Columbia
have passed such laws. Christina Jones explains:

> Hospitals and medical offices must do what is necessary
> to protect their patients from bacteria. Many hospitals use
> their cleaning budget as a place that they can cut corners,
> and this can be no more. I think it is very unfortunate that
> we have to legislate cleanliness in our hospital settings,
> but that is what we have to do. Several U.S. states and
> countries around the world have enacted laws requiring
> hospitals to disclose their infection rates, and many more
> have bills on the table. . . . I would love to think that hos-
> pitals would do this on their own, as good stewards of

their communities, but rising costs of all sorts have pushed them to save money where they can, and cleanliness is one area that they could trim the budget. . . . But what a shame to go into the hospital for a procedure to save your life, just to lose it to bacteria that you acquired during your hospital stay. This happens so frequently that I am sure the numbers would be absolutely shocking if they were revealed, and I am sure it is the reason that hospitals will not address this on their own.[64]

In an effort to curb the spread of infection, hospitals are installing dispensers of hand sanitizer and sinks with soap for both staff and visitors.

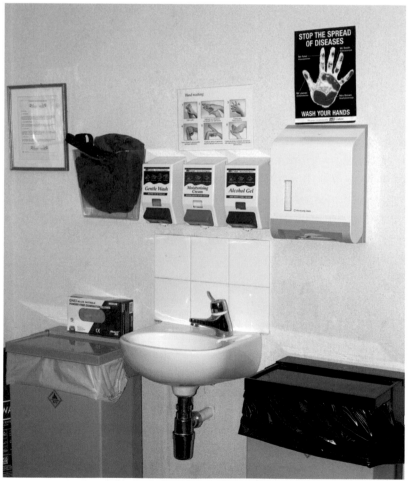

Another step that hospitals are taking is to install dispensers filled with alcohol based cleansers. These dispensers are placed throughout the building, and posted signs remind both staff and visitors to clean their hands. "I was impressed with the hospital I was in," Marilyn explains.

They had antiseptic gel dispensers inside and outside all the rooms. My daughter and my niece cleaned their hands before they came in to see me and when they left. I noticed the doctors and nurses did too. I think it was a good hospital. They were very conscientious about cleanliness. They cared about my health and safety. They didn't want me to get any sicker than I already was.[65]

To make sure that harried hospital workers make use of the cleansers, some hospitals are installing surveillance cameras. Others are using "spies." They are actually observers hired to see whether hospital employees clean their hands before and after treating patients. The information gathered by the observers is shared with hospital administrators and department heads, who then counsel health care providers who do not clean their hands.

Developing a Vaccine

Scientists at the University of Chicago are taking another approach to preventing new MRSA infections. They are working on a vaccine that will immunize individuals against MRSA. Vaccines create immunity to particular illnesses by exposing the immune system to a small dose of a greatly weakened or inactivated bacteria or virus. Such exposure stimulates the immune system to produce antibodies, which are naturally occurring proteins that recognize, lock onto, and destroy a specific germ. In the future, if MRSA invades a vaccinated person, the immune system will recognize the bacteria and quickly produce the appropriate antibodies to destroy it. Olaf Schneewind, chairman of microbiology at the University of Chicago, discusses the vaccine research:

This microbe's [MRSA] ability to acquire the tools it needs to protect itself from the drugs we use to treat it is legendary, which is why a vaccine has become such a high priority. One by one, this organism has learned to evade nearly all of our current antibiotics. So, generating protective immunity against invasive S. aureus has become an important goal.[66]

Because previous attempts at developing a vaccine did not produce a strong enough immune response to offer protection against MRSA, the scientists turned to a process known as reverse vaccinology. This involves sorting through the genome, or the genetic information, that MRSA carries to compile a list of specific surface proteins responsible for its virulence and, therefore, most likely to produce the strongest immune response. The scientists identified nineteen different proteins, which they injected into mice. They then measured the immune response that each protein generated. They came up with four proteins that produced the strongest immune response.

The next step was to divide the mice into five groups. Each of the first four groups was vaccinated with one of the identified proteins, but the fifth group was vaccinated with a combination of all four. Each group was then injected with a dose of MRSA calculated to kill 50 percent of the mice. One week later, 50 to 70 percent of the mice in the first four groups were still alive, depending on the particular protein they were administered. All of the mice that received the combination vaccine survived. The scientists are continuing to fine-tune the vaccine through animal testing. They hope to start clinical trials on humans soon.

Meanwhile, researchers at Harvard University Medical School in Boston are also working on developing a vaccine for MRSA, but they are employing a different tactic. Rather than using the bacteria's surface proteins to formulate a vaccine, they are focusing on a sugar called PNAG, which the bacteria produce. Natural exposure to PNAG does not cause a strong enough immune response to protect individuals from the bacteria. The scientists, however, discovered that they can chemically alter PNAG to produce different forms of the sugar, which

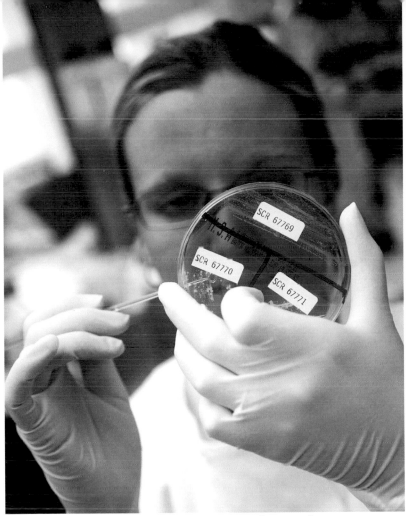
Scientists are studying the MRSA bacteria in hopes of creating a vaccine for the future.

induce a strong immune response in animal tests. "We now have a way to tip the balance for resistance to infection back towards humans by vaccination,"[67] explains researcher Gerald Pier. Human trials should begin by 2010. If the vaccine proves effective in trials, the scientists predict that the vaccine will be available in about ten years.

Viruses That Kill Bacteria

Whereas some scientists are working on developing a MRSA vaccine, other researchers are taking a different approach. They are looking at novel ways to destroy the bacteria. One interesting technique is bacteriophage therapy. Phages are viruses that prey on bacteria but do not harm body cells. Phages can be found in polluted water. According to medical journalist Amy Ellis Nutt:

> A phage is a virtual killing machine. Under a microscope it looks something like a NASA lunar lander. It consists of a 20-sided "head" atop a long, cylindrical neck that ends in a cone-shaped needle, or tail. It's the tail of the phage that makes contact with the bacterium, punching a hole through the cell's wall and acting like a syringe for the phage head to empty its genetic material into the center of the bacterium. Once in, the DNA overruns the place, promiscuously reproducing at a furious pace. "Daughter" phages multiply exponentially—100 in 30 minutes, 40,000 in the first hour, 4 billion in the second hour. Like a tire blowing out after being pumped with too much air, the cell, packed with new phage progeny, finally bursts, shredding in every direction.[68]

Different phages attack different types of bacteria. So far, phages specific to one hundred different bacteria, including MRSA, have been identified. Before patients can be treated

Phage therapy is one method researchers are using to destroy MRSA bacteria. A phage punctures the bacteria and releases its genetic material, which causes the bacteria to burst.

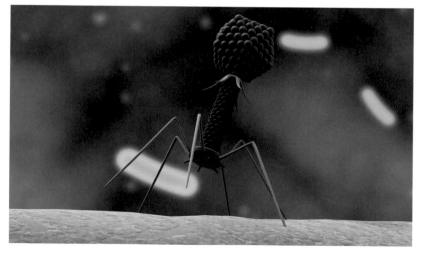

When to Take Antibiotics

Taking antibiotics unnecessarily increases the development of antibiotic-resistant bacteria. It is difficult for individuals to know when they should take antibiotics. Taking antibiotics for viral infections is inappropriate. Viruses cause these infections, and antibiotics have no effect on viruses. They do not keep viruses from spreading to other people, and they do not help infected individuals to feel better. Yet, according to the Centers for Disease Control and Prevention, millions of antibiotics are prescribed for viral infections each year, often as an unnecessary precautionary measure.

The flu, colds, chicken pox, measles, German measles, mumps, hepatitis, herpes, HIV/AIDS, shingles, polio, the stomach flu, and most respiratory infections, including a sore throat and bronchitis, are all viral illnesses. They should not be treated with antibiotics.

In contrast, bacterial pneumonia, strep throat, and some sinus and ear infections are caused by bacteria and do respond to antibiotic treatment.

with phages, however, phages must be collected from sewage or other sources. Viruses are applied to different bacterial cultures in order to determine the specificity of each collected phage. The mixtures are then placed in a centrifuge. If the bacteria are destroyed, the phages rise to the top of the sample.

Phage therapy has been used in eastern Europe for about eighty years. It was especially popular before antibiotics became readily available, and it is still commonly used in parts of the former Soviet Union. Because MRSA continues to develop resistance to more antibiotics, interest in bacteriophage therapy has increased in the rest of the world.

In 2008 researchers at the University of Strathclyde in Glasgow, Scotland, found that bacteriophages specific to MRSA bond to nylon. This means that the hospital dressing materials and nylon sutures used to stitch up patients during surgery could host the viruses. The researchers theorized that spreading the phages on sutures during surgery would help prevent infections, and dressing infected wounds with bandages treated with phages would better heal them. The researchers tested their theory in three Glasgow hospitals by applying phage-treated dressing to MRSA-infected wounds. Ninety-six percent of the infections were healed.

Although phage therapy is rarely used in the United States, its success abroad has sparked interest. If phage therapy continues to prove successful in Europe, it is possible that it will become a popular method of treating MRSA in the United States in the future.

Help from Maggots

Larval therapy is another old treatment that is being looked at as a way to destroy MRSA. For centuries maggots, or insect larvae, have been used to clean out wounds. When placed on a wound, they eat dead and infected tissue while leaving healthy tissue intact, essentially debriding a wound.

To keep the maggots from escaping, and so patients do not have to look at them, they are covered with dressing. Because they are so small, patients feel little pain as the maggots clean away dead and infected tissue. The sensation is often described as little scratches. After two or three days, the dressing containing the maggots is removed.

Professor Andrew Bolton of England's Manchester University, who is currently conducting research on the effect of larval therapy on MRSA infections, explains:

> Maggots are the world's smallest surgeons. In fact, they are better than surgeons—they are much cheaper and work 24 hours a day. They have been used since the Napoleonic wars and in the American civil war they found those who survived were the ones with maggots in their wounds: they kept them clean. They remove dead tissue and bacteria, leaving the healthy tissue to heal.[69]

Bolton and his team have successfully been using maggots to treat foot ulcers in diabetics at the Manchester Diabetes Center for ten years. Because the number of cases of patients coming into the center with ulcers infected with MRSA more than doubled between 2004 and 2007, the researchers decided to see whether larval therapy would have any effect on MRSA. The scientists applied maggots to the foot ulcers of thirteen MRSA-infected patients. The maggots completely destroyed twelve of the thirteen infections. Bolton called the results "very exciting." He explains:

> We have demonstrated for the first time the potential of larval therapy to eliminate MRSA infection of diabetic foot ulcers. . . . Larval treatment would offer the first non invasive risk-free treatment of this increasing problem and a safe and cost effective treatment, in contrast to the expensive and potentially toxic antibiotic remedies.[70]

Bolton and his team are currently conducting larger trials in an effort to prove the effectiveness of the therapy. At the same time, researchers at Swansea University in Wales have also been studying larval therapy. These scientists have isolated a

When placed on a wound, maggots eat dead and infected tissue while leaving healthy tissue intact.

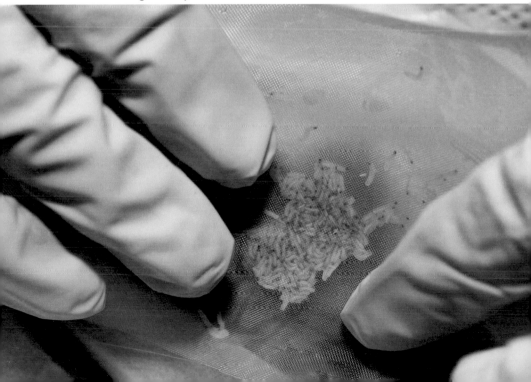

chemical called seraticin from maggots, which breaks down dead tissue and kills bacteria. These researchers are now working on a way to mass-produce seraticin. If they can do so, the chemical could be applied directly to MRSA infections.

Bathing in Bullfrog Protein

Still other scientists at St. Andrew's University in Scotland have come up with another interesting treatment. They combined ranalexin, a protein secreted by bullfrogs, with a chemical known as lysostaphin. Both substances are known to have antibacterial properties. The scientists theorized that when the two were combined they would be powerful enough to destroy MRSA. To test their theory, the researchers applied the compound to laboratory-cultured MRSA. In all cases, the mixture destroyed the bacteria. "Together the ranalexin and lysostaphin are very, very potent as any resistance has to overcome two hurdles. They kill the organism extremely quickly and effectively,"[71] explains microbiologist Peter Coote, who led the study.

Now that the researchers have shown that the mixture destroys MRSA cell colonies in laboratory tests, they are investigating whether it is equally effective as a topical application on medical devices such as catheters. If these experiments yield similar results, the mixture may be applied to indwelling medical devices in the future as a way to prevent and treat MRSA.

Green Clay's Healing Properties

In two separate studies, scientists at Arizona State University, Tempe, and at the University of Buffalo, New York, are investigating another new MRSA treatment—green clay. A French doctor named Line Brunet de Courssou used the clay, which is mined in France and is made from volcanic ash, to heal bacterial foot ulcers in patients in Africa. Brunet de Courssou's success sparked interest in the clay's healing properties.

In 2008 Arizona researchers divided MRSA cell cultures into two groups. They applied the clay to one group and then observed what happened over a twenty-four-hour time period. The other group served as a control and was, therefore, un-

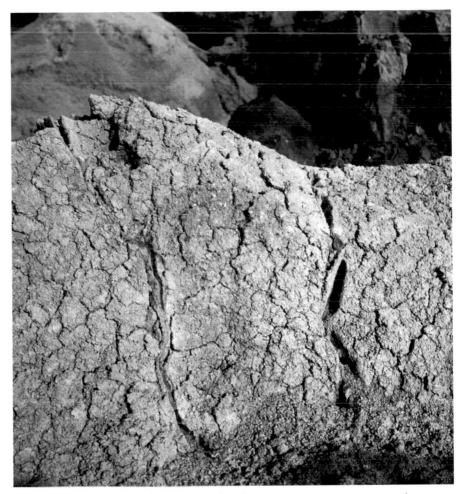

Green clay, like that on the French Atlantic coast, contains minerals that inhibit the bacteria's ability to function.

treated. The bacteria were eliminated in 99 percent of the samples treated with the clay. In the same time period, bacterial colonies in the control group grew by 45 percent. "It's fascinating," says researcher Shelley Haydel. "Here we are bridging geology, microbiology, cell biology. A year ago, I'd look at the clay and say, 'Well, it's just dirt.'"[72]

The scientists do not know how the clay destroys MRSA. They think it contains minerals that inhibit the bacteria's ability to function. Further research aimed at learning more about the clay and its effect on MRSA and other harmful bacteria is underway. If all goes well, it is likely that green clay will give health care providers yet another tool to combat MRSA in the future.

Until then, it is clear that scientists and health care experts are working hard to minimize the threat of MRSA. Innovative ways to destroy the bacteria and a possible vaccine offer new methods to control the bacteria. Ongoing measures to make hospitals safer are also having a positive impact. With all the work being done, it is possible that MRSA infections will become only a memory in the future.

Notes

Introduction: A Growing Problem

1. Quoted in Roxanna Sherwood and Vicki Mabrey, "MRSA 'Superbug' Becomes More Resistant," ABC News, March 5, 2008. http://abcnews.go.com/Health/Story?id=4393692&page =1.
2. Quoted in *Dallas News*, "U.S. Deaths from Staph 'Superbug' May Surpass AIDS Deaths," October 17, 2007. www.dallas news.com/sharedcontent/dws/news/dmn/stories/101707dn natstaph.17909.
3. Quoted in Christine Gorman, "Surviving the Killer Bug," Time.com, June 18, 2006. www.time.com/time/magazine /article/0,971,1205364,00.html.
4. Committee to Reduce Infection Deaths, "RID: The Cost of Infection." www.hospitalinfection.org/costofinfection.shtml.
5. Christina Jones, "An Open Letter to My Community," MRSA Resources, September 20, 2005. www.mrsaresources.com /an-open-letter-to-my-community/.

Chapter One: What Is MRSA?

6. Quoted in S. Williams, "Superbug: What Makes One Bacterium So Deadly," *Science News*, November 17, 2007, p. 307.
7. Bertha S. Ayi, *MRSA—Killer Bug*. Sioux City, IA: Lulu.com, 2007, p. 10.
8. Quoted in Sherwood and Mabrey, "MRSA 'Superbug' Becomes More Resistant."
9. Washington State Department of Health, "Living with MRSA," 2006, p. 4. www.3.doh.wa.gov/here/materials/PDFs /12_MTDSpage_E07L.pdf.
10. Quoted in Joyce Howard Price, "Hospitals' Hidden Danger," *Washington Times*, February 25, 2007. www.hospitalinfec tion.org/press/022507/washington_times.htm.

11. Quoted in MRSA Notes, "MRSA Post Laparoscopic Surgery." www.mrsanotes.com/mrsa-post-laparoscopic-surgery/#more-672.

12. Hernan R. Chang, *MRSA and Staphylococcal Infections*. Sioux City, IA: Lulu.com, 2006, p. 13.

13. Jessica Snyder Sachs, *Good Germs, Bad Germs*. New York: Hill and Wang, 2007, p. 125.

14. Ayi, *MRSA*, p. 31.

15. Quoted in Eric Nelson, "MRSA Information for Cops and Firefighters," MRSA Cop, April 7, 2008. http://mrsacop.blogspot.com/.

16. Quoted in CBS News, "Super-Resistant Superbugs," May 2, 2004. www.cbsnews.com/stories/2004/04/30/60minutes.

17. Quoted in Leslie Laurence, "Are You Safe from Superbugs?" *Ladies' Home Journal*, May 2007, p. 166.

Chapter Two: Symptoms, Diagnosis, and Treatment

18. Ayi, *MRSA*, p. 2.

19. Quoted in Britt Norlander, "Battling a Superbug: A Teen Athlete Struggles to Defeat Killer Germs," *Science World*, January 15, 2007, p. 10.

20. Quoted in MRSA Resources, "Marshall and Christina Jones, in College Station, Tx." www.mrsaresources.com/about/.

21. Christina Jones, "Marshall Jones: An MRSA Septicemia Survival Story," MRSA Resources, p. 2. www.mrsaresources.com/marshallsstory.pdf.

22. Quoted in ABC News, "'Superbug' MRSA Worries Doctors, Athletes," January, 13, 2005. http://rickylannetti.com/news articles/primetimelive.htm.

23. Quoted in MRSA Notes, "MRSA Post Laparoscopic Surgery."

24. Quoted in MRSA Notes, "A CA-MRSA Story," October 19, 2007. www.mrsanotes.com/A%20CA-MRSA%20Story/.

25. Ayi, *MRSA*, p. 22.

26. Quoted in Outzone TV, "Jack, Dating, HIV, and the Everyday Woman." http://blogs.outzonetv.com/runway/2007/jack_the_every_day_woman.php?page=2.

27. Quoted in Donna Wright, "Family Wants Schools to Protect Against MRSA," *Bradenton Herald*, April 22, 2008, p. 1.

28. Quoted in Steve Delsohn and Brian Franey, "MRSA Has Sidelined Careers, Even Caused Death," Kill CA-MRSA. www.killcamrsa.com/story1_sideline.html.

Chapter Three: Living with MRSA

29. Quoted in MRSA Notes, "A CA-MRSA Story."

30. Quoted in Sherwood and Mabrey, "MRSA 'Superbug' Becomes More Resistant."

31. Denise Rauff, "Denise Rauff's MRSA Story," MRSA Resources, November 12, 2006. www.mrsaresources.com/denise-rauffs-mrsa-story/.

32. John, interview with the author, Las Cruces, New Mexico, January 10, 2009.

33. Tony Field, "My Story for America," MRSA Resources. www.mrsaresources.com/tony-field-my-story-for-america/.

34. Michelle Wells, "MRSA Cleaning Tips from Michelle Wells," MRSA Notes, January 31, 2007. www.mrsanotes.com/mrsa-cleaning-tips-from-michelle-wells/.

35. Quoted in MRSA Resources, "Peg McQueary's MRSA Story." www.mrsaresources.com/peg-mcquearys-mrsa-story/.

36. Chang, *MRSA and Staphylococcal Infections*, p. 42.

37. Quoted in Sara Selis, "Not Your Father's MRSA: What You Need to Know—and Do—About Community-Associated MRSA," Consultant Live, November 8, 2007. www.consultantlive.com/display/article/10162/37699?pageNumber=3.

38. Quoted in Dale Keiger, "Drugs vs. Bugs," *Johns Hopkins Magazine*, February 2008. www.jhu.edu/jhumag/0208web drugbug.html.

39. Quoted in Patricia Kilday Hart, "Field of Nightmares," *Texas Monthly*, May 2006, p. 74.

40. Quoted in MRSA Survivors Network, "Survivor Stories." http://mrsasurvivors.org/id8.html.

41. Erin Zammett Ruddy, "Countdown to Decolonization: Hello Purell, Bye Bye MRSA!" Glamour.com, November 14, 2008. www.glamour.com/health-fitness/blogs/life-with-cancer/2008/11/countdown-to-decolonization-by.html.

42. Michelle Wells, "MRSA Cleaning Tips from Michelle Wells," MRSA Notes. www.mrsanotes.com/mrsa-cleaning-tips-from-michelle-wells/.

Chapter Four: Preventing MRSA Infections

43. Chuck Kimmel, "Handling MRSA," *Sports Medicine*, February/March 2006. www.athleticmanagement.com/2007/02/handling_mrsa.html.
44. Bronwyn Harris, "How to Prevent MRSA," How to Do Things.com. www.howtodothings.com/health-fitness/how-to-prevent-mrsa.
45. Mayo Clinic, "Hand Washing: A Simple Way to Prevent Infection." www.mayoclinic.com/health/hand-washing/HQ00407.
46. Wells, "MRSA Cleaning Tips from Michelle Wells."
47. Laurence, "Are You Safe from Superbugs?" p. 166.
48. Dwayne Jackson, "Stifle Staph," *Muscle & Fitness*, March 2008, p. 264.
49. Athletic Management, "Special Focus: Preventing MRSA Equipment Management." www.athleticmanagement.com/images/features/pdf/MRSAposter08-Equipment.pdf.
50. Bobbi Miller, "MRSA: How to Avoid Staph Infection in the Gym," Associated Content. www.associatedcontent.com/article/446820/mrsa_how_to_avoid_staph_infection_in.html?cat=50.
51. Quoted in Norlander, "Battling a Superbug," p. 10.
52. Quoted in Chris Cuomo, "Gym Germs Can Make You Sick," GymSoap.com, July 26, 2006. www.gymsoap.com/abcArticle1.php.
53. Wells, "MRSA Cleaning Tips from Michelle Wells."
54. Wells, "MRSA Cleaning Tips from Michelle Wells."
55. Betsy McCaughey, "Superbugs," Hudson Institute, September 27, 2005. www.hudson.org/index.cfm?fuseaction=publication_details&id=4991.
56. Committee to Reduce Infection Deaths, "15 Steps You Can Take to Reduce Your Risk of a Hospital Infection." www.hospitalinfection.org/protectyourself.shtml.
57. Quoted in Sarah Stewart, "Preventing Hospital Infections,"

KFOR.com, February 14, 2006. www.kfor.com/Global /story.asp?S–4503359.

58. Elizabeth Cohen, "Don't Let a Hospital Kill You," CNN.com. www.cnn.com/2008/HEALTH/05/01/ep.avoiding.infection/ index.html.

59. Quoted in *Second Opinion*, "Hospital Acquired Infection." www.pbs.org/secondopinion/episodes/hospitalacquiredinf ection/transcript/index.html.

Chapter Five: What the Future Holds

60. Betsy McCaughey, *Unnecessary Deaths: The Human and Financial Costs of Hospital Infections.* New York: Committee to Reduce Infection Deaths, 2008, p. 5. www.hospital infection.org/ridbooklet.pdf.

61. Quoted in Michael Barbella, *Drug Topics*, February 11, 2008, p. HSE1.

62. McCaughey, *Unnecessary Deaths*, p. 13.

63. Quoted in *Infection Control Today*, "More States Move to Require Hospitals to Screen Patients for MRSA," March 18, 2008. www.infectioncontroltoday.com/hotnews/requiring-mrsa-screening.html#.

64. Jones, "An Open Letter to My Community."

65. Marilyn, interview with the author, Las Cruces, New Mexico, January 24, 2009.

66. Quoted in University of Chicago News Office, "MRSA Vaccine Shows Promise in Mouse Study," October 3, 2006. www .news.uchicago.edu/releases/06/061030.mrsavaccine.shtml.

67. Quoted in Medical News Today, "Clue to MRSA Vaccine Is Bacteria's Sticky Glue," September 11, 2008. www.medicalnewstoday.com/articles/120997.php.

68. Amy Ellis Nutt, "Germs That Fight Germs," *Star Ledger*, December 9, 2003. www.nj.com/specialprojects/index.ssf? /specialprojects/plague/plague3.html.

69. Quoted in Debbie Andalo, "Maggots Feast on MRSA, Researchers Find," Guardian.co.uk, May 2, 2007. http:// education.guardian.co.uk/higher/research/story/0,,2070834, 00.html?gusrc=ticker-10.

70. Quoted in Andalo, "Maggots Feast on MRSA, Researchers Find."

71. Quoted in Metro.co.uk, "Bullfrogs Could Help Fight MRSA," April 30, 2007. www.metro.co.uk/news/article.html ?in_article_id=47315&in_page_id=34.

72. Quoted in David Gutierrez, "French Volcanic Clay Kills Antibiotic-Resistant Superbug," Natural News, April 15, 2008. www.naturalnews.com/023022.html.

Glossary

abscess: A bacterial infection of the skin that contains pus.

antibiotic resistance: The ability of a strain of bacteria to survive when exposed to drugs to which they were once susceptible.

antibiotics: Drugs that destroy bacteria.

bacteria: Single-cell microorganisms, which can cause disease.

bacteriophage: A virus that destroys bacteria.

boil: A bacterial infection of the skin that may or may not have pus.

catheter: A thin, flexible tube that is inserted into the body.

community-acquired MRSA (CA-MRSA): A MRSA infection that strikes otherwise healthy individuals who have not been hospitalized in the past year.

culture: A sample of bacteria grown in a laboratory; scientists then study the bacteria.

cytokines: Proteins produced by the immune system that initiate an inflammatory response.

debride: To remove dead and infected tissue in and around a wound.

epidemiologist: A medical expert who studies the transmission and control of contagious diseases.

hospital-acquired MRSA (HA-MRSA): A MRSA infection that is contracted in hospitals or other health care facilities, such as nursing homes.

indwelling medical device: Any medical device that is inserted into the body.

inflammation: The body's response to infection. It is characterized by heat, redness, tenderness, and swelling.

maggot: Insect larva.

methicillin-resistant *Staphylococcus aureus* (MRSA): A toxin-producing strain of *Staphylococcus aureus* that is resistant to multiple antibiotics.

pathogen: A germ.

***Staphylococcus aureus* (*S. aureus*, staph):** Toxin-producing bacteria that causes infections.

toxins: Poisons or proteins that act as poisons in the body.

vaccine: A medication that creates immunity to particular illnesses by exposing the immune system to a small dose of a greatly weakened bacteria or virus.

vancomycin: A powerful antibiotic that can usually destroy MRSA.

white blood cells: Cells whose job it is to attack and destroy foreign substances in the body.

Organizations to Contact

Centers for Disease Control and Prevention (CDC)
1600 Clifton Rd. NE, Atlanta, GA 30333
phone: (800) 311-3435
Web site: www.cdc.gov

The CDC's Web site offers information about how to prevent, treat, and live with MRSA.

Committee to Reduce Infection Deaths (RID)
185 East Eighty-Fifth St., Ste. 35B, New York, NY 10028
phone: (212) 369-3329
e-mail: betsymccaughey@hospitalinfections.org
Web site: www.hospitalinfections.org

RID is a nonprofit group dedicated to preventing hospital infections. It offers a wealth of information about MRSA and MRSA prevention.

National Institute of Allergy and Infectious Disease
6610 Rockledge Dr., MSC 6612, Bethesda, MD 20892
phone: (301) 496-5717
Web site: www.niaid.nih.gov

This agency offers information about various infectious diseases, including MRSA.

U.S. Food and Drug Administration
5600 Fisher Ln., Rockville, MD 20857
e-mail: webmail@oc.fda.gov
Web site: www.fda.gov

This government agency provides information about various bacteria and antibiotic resistance.

For Further Reading

Books

Bertha S. Ayi, *MRSA—Killer Bug*. Sioux City, IA: Lulu.com, 2007. A fairly simple adult book about MRSA.

Connie Goldsmith, *Superbugs Strike Back: When Antibiotics Fail*. Minneapolis: Twenty-First Century, 2006. A young adult book that looks at bacteria and how and why bacteria develop antibiotic resistance.

Patrick Guilfoile and Edward I. Alcamo, *Antibiotic Resistant Bacteria*. New York: Chelsea House, 2006. A young adult book that looks at different kinds of antibiotic-resistant bacteria.

Thomasine E. Lewis Tilden, *Help! What's Eating My Flesh?* New York: Scholastic, 2008. A young adult book consisting of case files of different bacterial infections, including MRSA. It contains lots of interesting pictures.

Periodicals

Patricia Kilday Hart, "Field of Nightmares," *Texas Monthly*, May 2006.

Dwayne Jackson, "Stifle Staph," *Muscle & Fitness*, March 2008.

Leslie Laurence, "Are You Safe from Superbugs?" *Ladies' Home Journal*, May 2007.

Britt Norlander, "Battling a Superbug: A Teen Athlete Struggles to Defeat Killer Germs," *Science World*, January 15, 2007.

S. Williams, "Superbug: What Makes One Bacterium So Deadly," *Science News*, November 17, 2007.

Internet Sources

Seattle Times, "A Special Report." http://seattletimes.nwsource.com/html/mrsa/.

Second Opinion, "Hospital Acquired Infection." www.pbs.org
/secondopinion/episodes/hospitalacquiredinfection/index.ht
ml.

Web Sites

MRSA Infection.org (www.mrsainfection.org/). This Web
site offers MRSA information, news, and many links.

MRSA Notes (www.mrsanotes.com/). A wealth of information
about MRSA is available on this site, including breaking
news and multiple links.

MRSA Resources (www.mrsaresources.com/). This Web site
provides information about MRSA, supports MRSA
awareness programs, and offers support to individuals with
MRSA.

MRSA Survivors Network (www.mrsasurvivors.org/index
.html). This Web site gives lots of information about MRSA,
including survivors' stories.

Index

Picture Credits

Cover: Image copyright Michael Taylor, 2009. Used under license from Shutterstock.com.

© CaptureItOne/Alamy, 45

© CNRI/PHOTOTAKE, Inc./Alamy, 22

© Custom Medical Stock Photo/Alamy, 52

© Helene Rogers/Alamy, 78

Image copyright Andrew Lever, 2009. Used under license from Shutterstock.com, 49

Image copyright JJJ, 2009. Used under license from Shutterstock.com, 59

Image copyright Larry St. Pierre, 2009. Used under license from Shutterstock.com, 26

Image copyright Ljupco Smokovski, 2009. Used under license from Shutterstock.com, 71

Image copyright Michael Taylor, 2009. Used under license from Shutterstock.com, 14

Image copyright Monkey Business Images, 2009. Used under license from Shutterstock.com, 35, 65

Image copyright Sean Nel, 2009. Used under license from Shutterstock.com, 0

Image copyright Sebastian Kaulitzki, 2009. Used under license from Shutterstock.com, 32, 82

Image copyright Sim Creative Art, 2009. Used under license from Shutterstock.com, 56

Image copyright Slowfish, 2009. Used under license from Shutterstock.com, 55

Image copyright spfotocz, 2009. Used under license from Shutterstock.com, 62

© Jim Mahoney/Dallas Morning News/Corbis, 66

Joe Raedle/Getty Images, 19

© Louise Murray/Alamy, 85

Mario Villafuerte/Getty Images, 74

© Richard Green/Alamy, 41

© Scott Camazine/PHOTOTAKE, Inc./Alamy, 29, 39

© Stephen Coll/Alamy, 87

Steve Zmina, 11

© Zak Waters/Alamy, 81

About the Author

Barbara Sheen is the author of more than forty books for young people. She lives with her family in New Mexico. In her spare time, she likes to swim, walk, exercise, garden, and cook.